Interprofessional Working for Health and Social Care

Community Health Care Series

Deborah Hennessy (editor)
Community Health Care Development

Ann Long (editor)
Interaction for Practice in Community Nursing

Carolyn Mason (editor)
Achieving Quality in Community Health Care Nursing

Jean McIntosh (editor)
Research Issues in Community Nursing

John Øvretveit, Peter Mathias and Tony Thompson (editors)
Interprofessional Working for Health and Social Care

Community Health Care Series
Series Standing Order ISBN 0-333-69328-0
(outside North America only)

You can receive future titles in this series as they are published by placing a standing order. Please contact your bookseller or, in the case of difficulty, write to us at the address below with your name and address, the title of the series and the ISBN quoted above.

Customer Services Department, Macmillan Distribution Ltd
Houndmills, Basingstoke, Hampshire RG21 6XS, England

Interprofessional Working for Health and Social Care

Edited by

JOHN ØVRETVEIT

PETER MATHIAS

AND

TONY THOMPSON

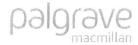

Published by
PALGRAVE
Houndmills, Basingstoke, Hampshire RG21 6XS and
175 Fifth Avenue, New York, N. Y. 10010
Companies and representatives throughout the world

PALGRAVE is the new global academic imprint of
St. Martin's Press LLC Scholarly and Reference Division and
Palgrave Publishers Ltd (formerly Macmillan Press Ltd).

ISBN 0–333–64553–7

This book is printed on paper suitable for recycling and
made from fully managed and sustained forest sources.

A catalogue record for this book is available
from the British Library.

Copy-edited and typeset by Povey–Edmondson
Tavistock and Rochdale, England

Transferred to digital printing 2002

Printed and bound in Great Britain by
Antony Rowe Ltd, Chippenham and Eastbourne

CONTENTS

LIST OF TABLES

The importance of interprofessional, multiprofessional and inter-sectoral working has been a live topic for debate within health and social services for well over a quarter of a century. Enquiry after enquiry on child abuse has pointed the finger at health and social work professionals for their failure to work cooperatively and collaboratively together and, as a result of this sin of omission, for their potential contribution to the death of a child.

More recently, reports published following mental health tragedies have been fiercely critical of professionals for the very same reasons.

Several of the recent Government policy documents have been written with collaboration between professionals and agencies as their focus. In 1978, the World Health Organisation in the famous Alma Ata Declaration strongly advocated for multiprofessional and multisectoral working and went one step further, by suggesting that the public should also be involved at every stage of the planning of health care. In more recent years, the British Government, through its Patient's Charter initiative and Local Voices, gave thumbs up to the public becoming partners in caring.

So far, we have done well on the rhetoric and less well on the action. Progress on interprofessional working has been patchy in the extreme: true patient participation is a long way off.

The reasons for this lack of progress are sometimes difficult to define, as there is so little research into the area. This book is therefore *timely and opportune*, as it helps to throw some light on a difficult subject. The fact that it is written by three professionals – a nurse, an expert in social work and a psychologist – with an impressive number of years of grassroots experience behind them, makes it all the more valuable. The book attempts to uncover some of the myths about interprofessional working. Like all of us, the authors believe in the intrinsic value of professionals and their agencies working effectively together. Including the users of the services as partners is perceived as not only a *desirable* but an *essential* goal. However, the authors sensibly acknowledge that when professionals operate under different management structures, have different paymasters, abide by different ethical and professional codes and sometimes have different end goals, interprofessional working is extremely difficult, although not impossible.

Working within the new internal market of health and social care further compounds the problem.

The imbalance of power which exists between professionals and service users – 'The professionals as a conspiracy against the laity' theory thus militating against the ideal of professional partnerships – is also well explored.

The case example of a community health team in action paints an excellent picture of just how complex the task is. The same can be said for the chapter on shared learning, which is presented warts and all.

However, the book also offers some solutions. The first lesson relates to our need to focus on the needs of the service user and not on the professional. The second lesson concerns the importance of learning together, yet acknowledging that, although we may come through different routes to our chosen specialist areas, we should embrace diversity and build on the many areas where we share common ground and which require similar competencies. The third lesson is that effective interprofessional working will not happen without a lot of effort on the part of all concerned, and even then not all of those efforts will have positive outcomes for either the service users or professionals. The fourth lesson concerns the importance of broadening our horizons, not only multiprofessionally and multisectorally but also Europe-wide.

This book should have wide appeal to everyone and anyone tackling the world of seamless and integrated care. It will be of particular interest to those professionals working or preparing to work in the field of health and social care. Managers or educationalists associated with those areas will find the book a useful addition to their libraries.

AINNA FAWCETT-HENESY
Acting Regional Adviser
Nursing and Midwifery
WHO Europe

Successive governments have indicated their commitment to enhancing the health of the nation and, in recent years, the focus of care delivery has shifted with escalating speed into the community. In so doing, it has become evident that community nurses and health visitors provide the focus for the promotion of health gain, and for the maintenance of positive health status for individuals, groups and local communities. Community nurses and health visitors are destined, therefore, to become leaders in the design, delivery and evaluation of effective health care interventions, informed by academic discovery, and advanced practice skills and competencies.

The changes that confront the contemporary community nursing practitioner are characterised by the diverse nature of the context within which community care is transacted, with an increasing emphasis on intersectoral co-operation, interprofessional collaboration, community action and development, and reduced reliance on the acute sector and residential care provision for longer-stay client groups.

The impact of change, pushed by a growing demand for flexible, high-quality services provided within local communities, will inevitably shape the NHS of the future. Resources have already been shifted to the community (although at a pace that is all too often criticised as being grossly inadequate to meet client need). Commissioners and providers are now required to demonstrate that the care they purchase and deliver is effective and responsive to the needs of local practice populations. To complement this, community nurses will be required to ensure that their activities make a significant impact on health gain for their practice population and, as such, must become seriously involved in structuring the political agenda that ultimately governs their practice environment.

In order for the community workforce to respond to these challenges, it will be necessary to ensure that community workers are equipped with the necessary skills and knowledge base to be able to function effectively in the 'new world of community health practice'. Nurses will be required to develop and change, drawing upon the very best of their past experience, and becoming increasingly reliant upon the production of research evidence to inform their future practice.

This series is aimed at practising community nurses and health visitors, their students, managers, professional colleagues and commissioners. It has been designed to provide a broad-ranging synthesis and analysis of the major areas of community activity, and to challenge models of traditional practice. The texts have been designed specifically to appeal to a range of professional and academic disciplines. Each volume will integrate contemporary research, recent literature and practice examples relating to the effective delivery of health and social care in the community. Community nurses and health visitors are encouraged towards critical exploration and, if necessary, to change their own contribution to health care delivery – at the same time as extending the scope and boundaries of their own practice.

Authors and contributors have been carefully selected. Whether they are nurses or social scientists (or both), their commitment to the further development and enrichment of health science (and nursing as an academic discipline in particular) is unquestionable. The authors all demonstrate knowledge, experience and excellence in curriculum design, and share a commitment to excellence in service delivery. The result is a distillation of a range of contemporary themes, practice examples and recommendations that aim to extend the working environment for practising community nurses and health visitors and, in so doing, improve the health status of their local consumer populations.

Interprofessional Working for Health and Social Care has been written by a nurse, an expert in social work and a clinical psychologist – with contributions from other professionals. It provides community practitioners with the opportunity for critical examination of multi-professional teamwork in the workplace with clients, carers and other agencies. The authors pay particular attention to interprofessional working across organisational boundaries, especially between health and social services. Drawing from an extensive literature on multidisciplinary teamwork, the authors provide a useful resource, assisting nurses to enhance their teamwork skills with the aim of equipping them to work effectively in a range of settings in the community. The book is firmly set within the context of societal change and encourages readers to reduce reliance on interprofessional methods of staff training and professional development. As such, it provides practitioners with the source material required to assist them in the provision of a 'seamless' and comprehensive service to clients and their carers on a range of community settings.

DAVID SINES
University of Ulster, Belfast

xii

Simon Biggs, BSc, PhD, AFBPsS, CQSW, is Senior Lecturer in Social Policy at the University of Keele, Staffordshire.

Margaret Coats, BSc, is Director of the Occupational Standards Council for Health and Social Care, UK.

Peter Mathias, BSc, MA, PhD, is Director of the Joint Awarding Bodies (a joint arrangement between CCETSW and the City and Guilds London Institute). He has a varied experience in social care practice, research and training.

Lindsay Mitchell is Director of PRIME Research and Development Ltd. She has been involved in research and development, relating particularly to the care sector, for many years.

John Øvretveit, BSc, MPhil, PhD, CPsychol, MHSM, is Professor of Health Policy and Management, and Director of the Nordic Quality Network, Nordic School of Public Health, Gothenburg, Sweden. His previous post was that of Director of the Health and Social Services Management Programme at Brunel University, UK.

Ruth Prime BA, Certificate in Social Work, was formerly Social Services Inspector at the Department of Health and Social Services.

Tony Thompson, MA, BEd, RMN, RNMH, DN, CertEd, RNT, is Director of Practice Development at the Ashworth Centre, Ashworth Hospital, Liverpool. His previous post was that of ENB Adviser in Mental Health and Learning Disabilities.

Jenny Weinstein, BPhil (Social Work), MSc, is Social Work Education Adviser at the Central Council for Education and Training in Social Work (CCETSW). She is currently involved in a range of projects to promote, develop and evaluate interprofessional education and to involve users in the planning, delivery and monitoring of training.

As professional practitioners, we like to think that the success of health and social care interventions are due to our own abilities. When the client or patient makes no progress, we often think that it is because we lack the skills, knowledge or experience to help them. In the past the individual professional's skills may have been the main determinant of good or bad care – but is this still the case? We have been trained in this 'professional-centric' view of the world, and our work-places and our professional associations uphold what we call the 'myth of the omnipotence of the individual practitioner'.

This myth is helpful for some clients and patients at certain times. A day before surgery, or when recovering from a heart attack, or when going through a period of intolerable anxiety – at these times it helps to believe that the practitioner is capable of anything and completely to be trusted. Professions have worked for many years to create and sustain this myth, not just to secure lucrative markets, but also because the myth can assist in helping people.

Yet the reality of modern health and social services is that the care we get depends as much on how professionals work with each other as on their individual competence within their own field of expertise. Our belief in the skill of the surgeon and her actual competence is important, but so also is her ability to work with other professionals in the operating room, and with many others in diagnostics, therapeutics and in the wards. In the traditional pre-serve of the lone solo practitioner – in primary and community care settings – the ability of the family doctor, the community nurse the therapist and others to help a person depends on their knowledge of and ability to work with other professionals.

Not only does the care we get depend on interprofessional working, so do the costs of what we get. As finance reduces, and as more people pay for more elements of their care directly, the cost of care is as important as the quality of care. Many services can no longer afford the duplication, mistakes and delays which can occur when professions do not work together. Services have to look more closely at skill-mix and consider whether practitioners can do work which other professions have traditionally done. Cross-training and flexible working are becoming more widespread. We are more aware that practitioners in other countries do different tasks and that there is nothing sacred in current work boundaries. Many services have also found that improving interprofessional working has both lowered costs, and increased quality.

This is not to devalue the skill and knowledge of professional practitioners, rather it is to suggest that certain skills and knowledge are becoming more important. In addition to profession-specific competency, practitioners in modern health and social services need knowledge of what other professionals can and cannot do, and the skills to work with them. As we show in this book, these competences are increasingly needed by practitioners in Europe and beyond, and there are a number of initiatives now in progress for developing these competences.

THE BOOK

In short, as well as competent practitioners we need competent systems, and a central feature of a competent system is effective interprofessional working. This is a book about interprofessional working written by different professionals. Each worked as a practitioner with other professions before taking up training and development roles, helping to develop different aspects of inter-professional working. The book aims to help practitioners to reassess how they work with other professionals, and to show ways in which they and managers can improve interprofessional working, with a realistic knowledge of the difficulties and advantages of doing so.

A broad subject defined

Interprofessional working is a broader subject than multidisciplinary teamwork. It is defined as 'how two or more people from different professions communicate and cooperate to achieve a common goal'. The goal is usually a positive outcome for a patient or a client; for example stabilising diabetes, return to previous mobility, or living independently. Interprofessional working can range from, at one extreme, making a referral to another professional, through increasing 'closeness' of working to making a joint assessment, working together as co-therapists, or working as an operating-room team.

The subject of interprofessional working is also broader than describing how practitioners work together to help patients or

2

clients. It describes how professionals work together to undertake management and planning tasks, which benefit a group of patients or contribute to the running and planning of service organisations. Examples of formal groups are management teams, project teams, planning teams, training teams, multidisciplinary audit groups and quality groups. Examples of tasks include formulating a procedure for referrals and assessments to be followed by many professions, deciding a plan to reduce higher than average length of stay, deciding a joint health and social services training programme, creating a purchasing plan for a community care plan, agreeing a care management model, and working in a quality group to reduce the rate of readmissions.

A focus on practitioners

Just from this definition we can see that interprofessional working is the predominant way of working in health and social services and Chapter 9 gives a fuller discussion of the concept. We have limited the scope of this book to concentrate on interprofessional working at the level of patient or client care and between 'direct patient/client contact' or 'clinical' practitioners. Examples are how family doctors (GPs or primary care physicians), community nurses, social workers and therapists work together, whether or not each is a member of a primary care team; how primary care practitioners work with secondary care practitioners or specialists in health and social services who are based in a hospital or in a community setting; and how specialists work with each other, for example in community networks or in teams such as a rehabilitation team, a surgical team, a community mental health or learning disability team, or a specialist team for children, families or older people.

Our focus is on interprofessional working in two types of situations. The first is around the care of an individual patient or client, sometimes involving a relative or other informal carer. We can describe the practitioners involved as 'the patient's or client's team'. Where they do not meet, and talk, we have 'relay' teams. In these each practitioner makes their contribution in succession, passing the client to the next practitioner in a chain of care. Here there is a need for 'coordination-for-continuity' to ensure a seamless care episode. For some clients and patients needing the help of many practitioners at one time, interprofessional working needs to be coordinated to ensure that each person's efforts have a mutually-reinforcing effect, or 'coordination for care synergy'. One method

3

for ensuring both types of coordination is for one person to act as a coordinator to ensure that each practitioner knows what the others are doing, or have done, and to adjust their efforts accordingly. This coordination role takes many different forms and is given many different names, more usually a care- or case manager.

The second situation is where the same practitioners regularly work together serving the same types of patients or clients. Examples are formal multiprofessional teams, or less-integrated networks as in some primary care settings. Here we are concerned with practitioner coordination in a different sense: as well as coordination in the care of one patient or client, we are concerned with routine coordination mechanisms which apply in many cases, and with agreed procedures and communication systems. Interprofessional working is different in these two situations. At one extreme, in the patient's or client's team, practitioners may never meet and may only communicate through written referral forms or records. At the other extreme, in some fully-integrated formal teams such as stroke rehabilitation teams, practitioners may always work with the same practitioners when they care for different patients or clients. Patient and practitioner coordination is easier in formal teams than in temporary patient or client teams, but practitioners need to be able to work with other professions in both situations. Interprofessional working in both situations is increasing – with practitioners with whom we only have infrequent contact, and with practitioners we work with regularly in a formal multiprofessional team.

Our focus in the book, then, is on how practitioners work together now and in the future. We consider practical details of day-to-day working and of teamwork, and we look at how this will change with developments in the UK and in Europe. We look at ways of improving interprofessional working at the level of daily practice, and through new types of training initiatives. We pay particular attention to interprofessional working across organisational boundaries, especially between health and social services. There are three reasons for our focus on interprofessional working at the practice level. First, it is what we know about and have worked on in different ways for all of our professional lives. Second, we are convinced of the importance of the subject to people's wellbeing and to the future of health and social services. Third, whilst there is a growing body of literature on multidisciplinary teams, we felt that there are issues to be addressed and work we wanted to share concerning the wider subject of interprofessional working which are relevant in many different countries.

4

CHAPTERS OF THE BOOK

Day-to-day interprofessional working

Although interprofessional working is a broader subject than multi-professional teams, a large amount of interprofessional working is organised within multidisciplinary teams. We see in Chapter 1 that 'multidisciplinary' or 'multiprofessional' team is a term used to describe a variety of different working arrangements. A team is 'a bounded group of people with a common purpose and a formal or informal organisation'. Interprofessional working occurs within teams, as well as between team members and practitioners outside of the team. A problem in designing and improving teams is that people use the same word to describe different types of teams. We need to be able to describe different types of teams and types of interprofessional working for a number of purposes: to help new practitioners to understand how a team works, to compare different people's ideas about what type of team to create, to work out where to make improvements, and to do research and evaluation into which types are most effective or least costly in different settings for different clients or patients (Øvretveit, 1996).

Chapter 1 gives four ways to describe a team: in terms of (i) degree of integration; (ii) membership; (iii) client pathway and decision-making; and (iv) in terms of management structure. Using these four aspects of a team we can describe a particular team and distinguish it from another team or type of team. The chapter shows the ways in which teams within different sectors differ from each other and from teams in other sectors. We see how many primary health care teams are completely different from each other and that most generalisations about 'the' primary health care team are misleading. We see the variety of types of community and hospital teams and consider how to improve interprofessional working in each.

Chapter 2 will be of most interest to managers but it will also help practitioners understand that many causes of poor cooperation are not personal failings but poor planning and management. It continues the theme of multiprofessional teamwork by outlining principles and concepts for setting up and managing a team. Many teams 'happen' by a combination of circumstances such as 'lucky' finance becoming available, the coincidence of a building becoming empty, and a manager convinced of the idea. Few are planned and fewer are set up on the basis of an assessment of people's needs. The result is predictable problems which some teams do not survive. Chapter 2 argues against the anarchist sink-or-swim model of team formation and management. It describes a way of combining a rational approach to team planning and management with a flexible and pragmatic programme of team development.

It is a common saying that if practitioners are 'left to get on with it', they will forge links and develop interprofessional working in appropriate and effective ways – that the problem is managers or too many reorganisations. This may or may not be true and much depends on practitioner training and past experiences. It is true, however, that interprofessional working is more difficult when practitioners work for different organisations, especially health and social services. Working across professional service and agency boundaries is one of the themes of Chapter 3, which gives a practical description of the details of interprofessional working in one community mental health centre. This case example illustrates in a practical way some of the issues covered in other chapters: how to assess needs and work together with different professional languages, how to shift from profession-services to more interprofessional working, and how to combine team leadership with profession- and agency- management structures.

Chapter 4 moves from team organisation to team-client or team-patient relations. It considers how increasing patient and client-power affects how professions work together. It describes what we mean by patient involvement and client participation and looks at the trends which are changing the traditional balance of power between professionals and patients or clients. The chapter gives a framework for auditing and improving patient or client participation in decision-making, and then assesses how these changes are affecting interprofessional working. It proposes that greater participation calls for closer interprofessional working, and speculates whether close-knit multidisciplinary teams are also better at involving patients and clients in key decisions in their treatment and care.

Training and preparation for interprofessional working

The next part of the book turns to how to train and prepare people for interprofessional work. As well as describing the general issues, it draws lessons from shared and joint-learning initiatives.

Chapter 5 looks at trends and changes in education in the UK. It argues that opportunities for interdisciplinary and interprofessional experience and learning should be consciously and deliberately built

6

into education for practitioners before, during and after their professional education for qualification. It shows how recent initiatives in the development of vocational education can help to promote interprofessional, cross-discipline or inter-agency perspectives.

Chapter 6 returns to the question of participation and describes how people who use a service can help to get unified and integrated programmes of health and social care. It looks at the implications of recent developments in community care and at the various purposes of interprofessional training.

Chapter 7 gives our second care example by describing a project which ran between 1990 and 1995 to encourage the joint training of practice teachers and clinical supervisors in nursing, occupational therapy and social work. The chapter gives a useful model for those interested in organising joint training programmes and illustrates the changes in the roles and status of health care professionals, the moving boundaries between them and the interface between those changes and current developments in professional education and training.

The future of interprofessional working

The third part of the book turns to the future of interprofessional working. It considers the impact on professions and interprofessional working of different national, European and international initiatives.

Chapter 8 looks at issues in interprofessional working through the perspective of the' functional map of health and social care'. The functional map, developed by the UK's Occupational Standards Council for Health and Social Care, gives an overview of all the work roles in the sector in an integrated and coherent way. It does so by looking at how those who work in the sector aim to meet the needs of service users, whatever their professional background and training and however this is carried out by a single profession or through interprofessional work. The map can be used as a starting point to thinking about interprofessional working and to inform the development of interprofessional qualifications.

Chapter 9 outlines recent social policy initiatives on interprofessionalism, its direction and some of the implications. It examines terms and concepts in relation to both the 1989 Children Act and the 1990 NHS and Community Care Act. The chapter cautions against an uncritical acceptance of interprofessional work as a

7

'good thing', gives ideas about how interprofessionalism can lead to an improved service, and argues that future efforts towards interprofessional collaboration must build on the strengths of management coordination, professional expertise and increased userparticipation which were covered in earlier chapters. Initiatives of the World Health Organisation (WHO) and the European Union will have an increasing impact in the coming years. In Chapter 10 we identify the broad shape of the influences likely to emerge from the two organisations and examine, in some detail, European Vocational Policies and the World Health Organisation's *Health for All* targets. We propose that the overall challenge is to combine the different components of the various policies and targets into cohesive programmes of work, each of which stimulates, involves and gives incentives to the public, private and voluntary sectors at local, national and international levels and to the professions in their progress towards the achievement of the goals.

We have taken a deliberately practical and future oriented approach in this book, and we look forward to further participation in practice and debates about:

● the purpose, organisation and methods of interprofessional working;
● the contribution of academic, professional and vocational education to health and social care;
● the work of British Nordic and European institutions concerned with policies and targets for health and social care and for intersectoral working.

Reference

Øvretveit, J. (1996) *Evaluation: An introduction to evaluation of health treatments, services and policies*, The Nordic School of Public Health, Goteborg, Sweden.

8

CHAPTER ONE

How to Describe Interprofessional Working

John Øvretveit

INTRODUCTION

'Why do you all ask me that same question – don't you people talk to each other?' We have all had clients say this, and many of us have explained it as a problem of 'bureaucracy' or 'communications' – the two explanations for problems which most people seem to accept. But when we and the other people whom the client has been seeing are all part of one team, we question what type of team we are in and how effective it is.

We have all joined a team, only to discover it was not the type of team which we imagined. We remember that team members emphasised how good and close the teamwork was, but said little more. The operational policy seemed to explain it all, but after a while we saw the gaps in the policy and noticed that people do not follow it. They all did their own thing, and some did not even come to the team meetings. In fact, many seemed to be members of other teams. Should we start asking questions, or start to contribute to 'the myth of the team'? Perhaps, in time, we will learn to see the emperor's clothes.

Look hard and you will find that many multidisciplinary teams are no such thing, especially in primary care (Jones, 1992). But you then have to recognise that you have assumptions about what a team should be. Sometimes 'multidisciplinary team' is a name describing all the people who work in a particular service – there has never been a meeting and many people in the team do not know who the others are. The name 'team' may also be given to an infrequent meeting of a variety of different people, with bases and loyalties elsewhere. Such meetings may in fact be very useful, but should we use the word team to describe both this meeting and a group of people who work together full-time with agreed objectives, and who share the same base and secretaries?

Over the last fifteen years I have worked with 134 groups each of which called themselves a multidisciplinary team. I have come to recognise that I must start work without making assumptions about what the group is (indeed whether there is a group in the usual sense) and about how it works. The best approach is to discover the different types of interprofessional working and communications which exist. For example, certain people regularly attend a weekly meeting to take clients onto their caseload. The group also has a common referral form which they all ask referrers to use. There are agreed conventions for record keeping, and a meeting chairperson. Add these different, agreed and sometimes written arrangements together and you have one type of team.

However there are some arrangements which are more common where professions seek to work more closely together. This chapter describes these arrangements later. It shows how groups adopt very similar combinations of arrangements, and that in these instances we can talk about a 'type' of team which is different to another type which has a different set of arrangements.

Concepts for describing teams

Much confusion and many problems arise from the use of the term multidisciplinary team to describe many different types of arrangements. This is one reason why this book prefers to use the term interprofessional working, and to consider different type of arrangements for different purposes. In order to design or improve interprofessional working arrangements we need to be able to distinguish and describe different types of team, and consider which type is best suited to the needs of a particular client group and the resources available. The purpose of this chapter is to give ways to describe different types of interprofessional working. For readers who are in a team, this can help you to understand what type of team you are in and what type of team your team could become. For readers setting-up teams, the descriptive framework helps to decide what type of team to establish. Researchers will find that the ways of describing and categorising a team help to evaluate teamwork and to discover which type is most effective for certain purposes.

This chapter presents the four ways of describing and defining a team which I have found most useful for research and for team development purposes. The first is in terms of 'degree of integration', which is a way of describing the degree of closeness of working between professions. The second is in terms of 'membership' of a permanent work group – who is and is not a member of the team, and what membership means. The third is in terms of process, described by defining a 'client pathway' through the team and noting how certain decisions are made about who does what. The fourth is in terms of management – how the team is led and how practitioners are managed.

We will concentrate on groups of practitioners from different professions serving a population of patients or clients, rather than on the group of people at any one time serving one person (a patient's or client's team or a 'relay team'). Examples of the former are primary health care teams, teams in hospital services, rehabilitation teams, community mental health teams, learning disability teams, child and family teams, drugs and alcohol teams and teams for older people.

INTEGRATION

The first way of describing a team is in terms of the degree of integration. Teams vary in terms of how the team influences an individual team member's work decisions. In some the team meeting or policy (if one exists) has a limited influence, such as on whether to take on a client. In others, the team may strongly influence the details of the practitioner's clinical decisions, and their own-profession manager (if they have one) has no influence.

The best way to explain the concept of 'degree of integration' is to describe two ends of a continuum. At one end is a loose-knit team called a 'network'. Some people would not call a network a team at all, because membership changes and is voluntary. At the other extreme is a closely integrated team, where team members' workload and clinical decisions are governed by a multidisciplinary team policy and by decisions made at the team meeting. This closeness of integration is because the group is collectively accountable for serving a population.

11

Network meeting teams

In network teams (Figure 1.1), practitioners are organised in professional services and managed by their profession-manager. People are referred to each profession's service entry point and each professional service has its own policies, priorities and procedures. The network is made up of practitioners who serve the same 'type' of clients or patients, either because they have the same type of needs or come from the same area. Practitioners use the network or the network meeting to cross-refer, or arrange work-in-parallel. The more that practitioners have in common (for example the same area or types of patients), then the more efficient it is for them to meet regularly to cross-refer. It saves their time and the patient's time for them to bring referrals to the meeting to pass on to others, or to check if it is appropriate to make a referral to others.

In addition, practitioners may use network meetings to organise work which they share with other practitioners (for example with a patient or a carers' group); to agree how to coordinate a complex care programme for a person served by members of the network; to discuss cases in more depth; or to organise project work or

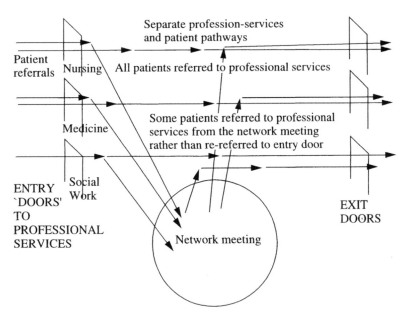

Figure 1.1   A network meeting team

12

formulate shared views to represent to higher authorities. Attendance at meetings and participation in the network is voluntary and informal, and is easily disrupted by changes such as sickness, short-staffing, or reorganisations in agencies or in each professional service. Examples of a network team are most primary health care teams, and some mental health, learning disabilities, child care and other specialist teams, especially where practitioners have different employing agencies.

Integrated interprofessional team

At the other end of the continuum is the integrated team (Figure 1.2). In this type of team there is a 'one door entry' to all of the profession's services and one team leader, although practitioners often also have senior professional advisors. There is an agreed set of objectives and priorities and an operational policy with procedures governing all members of the team. Full integration (for example one team manager for all) is not possible where team members are employed by different agencies, because team members remain accountable to their different employers. There is often a 'core' integrated team, with 'associates' who are members of other professional services (a hybrid network/integrated team). There are many variations of this type of team according to how the team influences members' work-management and clinical decisions, as we consider later when looking at client/patient pathways.

The above describes two ends of the continuum. We can place a team on this continuum according to which practitioner decisions the team influences and how strongly the team influences these decisions (Øvretveit, 1993). This continuum refers to formal influ-

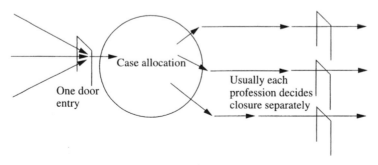

Figure 1.2   An integrated interprofessional team

13

ences. These to a large extent account for the experience we have of how closely we work with other professions in a group and how integrated the team is. However, we may work with others in a network where there is close cooperation, and in fact this group may feel more integrated than a multidisciplinary team which has many formal integration arrangements. The point is that the continuum of integration accounts for much, but not all, of the experience of 'closeness' of interprofessional working.

The 'collective responsibility team' and the 'coordinated profession team'

Integration as described above relates to the question of whether the team is viewed as a separate accountable service in its own right, which is another aspect of integration. The distinction between a collective responsibility team and a coordinated profession team is fundamental to clarifying what type of team a particular team is supposed to be, and to working through misunderstandings (Øvretveit, 1993). Most networks are coordinated profession teams (CPTs), defined here as 'referral and communication meetings for separately organised and accountable professional services'. Fully-integrated teams are collective responsibility teams (CRTs) – 'teams in which members are accountable as a group for pooling and using their collective resources in the best way to meet the most pressing special needs of the population they serve'. This does not mean that in CRTs members are accountable as a group for any clinical decisions, just for how they allocate their collective resources in a management sense. In any team, each individual member is always professionally accountable for their own case work and omissions.

In CPTs, different professions have their own formally-agreed priorities and are financed and managed to provide specific services. They meet to cross-refer and are influenced by the ideas of other professions, but they are essentially self-directing and accountable separately to their profession-managers and to those paying for how they use their resources. In CRTs, the team as a whole has to manage its collective resource to serve a population, and the team is financed as an entity in its own right. Even part-time members of the team, in their 'team time', must work to the collective priorities of the team and consider their time as a team resource. They share responsibility with the others for working out how to serve a priority client referred to the team – they cannot opt out because that type of client or need is not a priority for their profession or

14

agency. On the other hand, members of such teams cannot undertake work with a client or patient which they are not competent to do, because they remain accountable as individual professionals for their case work. If the team is not staffed properly for the needs it has to meet, there can be conflicts between a practitioner's professional accountability and their 'collective resource responsibility', as we see in Chapter 2.

Being a member of a collective responsibility team means that your day-to-day decisions are influenced by the team. This is how the team makes sure that the team resources – which includes your time – are used to the best effect. If the influence results in your skills not being used, then something is wrong – but it is a team issue. In some teams it is not always clear whether some or all members share a collective responsibility, even if they feel that they do. Where members have enjoyed a high degree of autonomy in the past, they are understandably reluctant to give up valued or familiar work in order to take on work because it is a team priority, especially if others in the team are not doing so. Getting the right balance between team control over resources and member autonomy is an issue we touch on below, and deal with more fully in the next chapter on team flexibility.

It is the job of managers to make this collective responsibility clear, if that is what is intended for the team. Often it is only by recognising that the team is not serving the clients most in need that leads managers to confront this issue. Each profession or employment group is so tied up meeting their specific responsibilities that no one has time left to serve certain clients. The problem is less severe in teams that have the right mix and amount of professions for the needs of the community – each profession following their own priorities results in a reasonable match to needs. But needs and membership change, and needs have to be matched to resources week-to-week, as well as over the longer term.

Managers must clarify whether a team is for client-coordination only, or for 'collective service' (what I have called elsewhere, 'accountable service-provision teams' (Øvretveit, 1986)), or for both. Managers have to change the responsibilities of their staff and change staff management if their staff are to contribute properly to a collective-service-provision team. If managers do not, then the agency and professional responsibilities will always come before the team's collective responsibility to serve a population. For example, social workers employed by a social service department are paid to carry out department policies and priorities.

15

They may be assigned to serve a client group in a locality, but they provide a social work service according to their department policies and priorities. If their manager does not modify their responsibilities to make it possible to take part in providing a collective service, then it is likely that their departmental responsibilities will take up so much of their time that they cannot take on clients that are a team priority, or even contribute to multidisciplinary case discussions.

TEAM MEMBERSHIP

The second way of describing a team is in terms of membership. Membership defines a group's boundaries. A network is a fluid arrangement where attendance at meetings is voluntary, and practitioners are either members of profession-teams or other teams, or independent practitioners. Their loyalty is usually elsewhere. In a fast-changing situation, and for some purposes, an open network with changing attenders is the most appropriate mechanism for communication and cooperation between agencies and professions.

The moment we talk of network 'membership' we imply less fluidity and more permanence and stability. We begin to think of a group with regular attenders and the concepts of attender's obligations to the group and of rights and commitment begins to arise. The question of team membership often arises when a group is evolving from a network into a formal team. Agreeing membership is a way of drawing boundaries around the group. In the early stages everyone is a member and no distinctions are made. It threatens the weak bonds holding the group together to make distinctions. Later, when important decisions have to be made, for example about priorities or whether to have self-referral or crisis intervention, the meaning of membership becomes more important. Is it right that people who are not affected by the decision, or who often do not come to meetings, have an equal vote to those whose working week will be profoundly affected by the decision? Are those not affected in fact real members of the group?

If everyone is a team member then there is no team, or the team is a very general entity and the word team is used to signal some similarity between members, but nothing else. Yet to exclude some people from team membership would be wrong. For instance, therapists or physicians may only be able to give part of their working week to the group and should be considered full members.

Many groups avoid facing up to the question of membership because it means confronting some of the key underlying questions of team structure and facing difficult decisions. It reveals differences of view about the nature of the group and about group purpose, differences which threaten to break up the weak integration which has been achieved in the team's evolution.

Clarifying membership often marks a transition from an informal loose-knit group to a more formal and organised team. It happens as a result of, or as part of, a process of clarifying the purpose of the group. This transition is helped by being able to assign different categories of membership, so as to recognise differences in the group and keep valued contributors. The most common membership distinction is between 'core' and 'associate' (or extended team), usually meaning full-time in the team or part-time (Øvretveit, 1993). This chapter follows this usage, but it is important to recognise that the terms core and associate can also refer to one or more of the types of membership listed below, and have nothing to do with 'commitment to the team'.

'Core,' can mean:	*'Associate,' can mean:*
Full-time in a team	Part-time in a team
All who are governed by the team policy	Those not governed by the team policy
All those managed by the team leader	Those with managers outside of the team
Formal voting rights	No voting rights on team decisions

A second membership question is which mix of different professions and other staff should be in the team and how many of each. In some instances there is a choice, for example when planners and managers are designing a new team. Here it is possible to start from an analysis of the type and amount of different client or patient needs; then to decide the mix and amount of different professions and level of skill which would be necessary to meet the most pressing needs. If the planners get it right then the team will find that they are not short of the right skills for the demands placed on them – they can get a good match between the individual client's need and the skills in the team.

Often, however, team membership is the result of historic staffing decisions and arbitrary fate. Managers work with what they have and, if they are able, change professions and staff grades when

17

people leave in order to get a better match between the demands on the team and the range of skills available. In the past, team membership has often been decided by profession-managers pressing for members of their profession to be in the team, regardless of whether it leads to the right overall balance of skills in the team (Hunter and Wistow, 1989). In the future, team managers may have more flexibility to appoint or contract-in people with the skills that are needed, regardless of their professional background. Will team managers have the expertise to know which skills are required for the demands to be placed on a team in the next two years?

A third aspect of membership is the more personal aspects of each member: their skills apart from profession-specific skills, their experience, status and seniority. In the same way as there is a tendency to avoid defining membership in developing teams, there is also a tendency to avoid recognising real and important seniority and status differences between team members. This observation is based on experience working with a number of teams. If this phenomenon is widespread, it may be worth examining hypotheses about why it happens. One hypothesis is that recognising these differences within a team may undermine a tentative consensus about purpose which is essential to holding the group together. Another is that team members fear that recognising payment and status differences may release destructive feelings of jealousy and envy which cannot be contained by the fragile mechanisms which exist within the team. A third is that teams which wish to establish participatory and more equal relations with clients also stress equality and democracy within the team.

It is curious that some teams find it easy to recognise sex and race differences in a team and try to appoint new members to ensure the right balance, yet deny differences in experience, status and seniority. I will not speculate further as to the reason for this, but simply note that not recognising these differences devalues the skills and many years' experience of senior team members. These differences must be recognised in order to make effective arrangements for:

- client–practitioner matching: a client with complex and acute problems will usually need the skills and knowledge of a more senior and experienced practitioner.
- team members' development: one of the best ways to learn is 'by doing', with expert oversight. Teams can ensure both that their members develop and that they meet client demands by arranging for more experienced team members to supervise other team

members. This is especially important if junior team members do not have easy access to more senior members of their own profession. Arranging cross-professional supervision is also a way of developing interprofessional understanding and cooperation.

A fourth aspect of membership is the role of members, the work that they do, and their autonomy. We consider these issues below when looking at team management structures, and in the next chapter when looking at operational policies and team flexibility.

TEAM PROCESS: CLIENT PATHWAYS AND DECISION-MAKING

A third way of describing a team is in terms of the stages a patient or client passes through on their journey to and through a team, and in terms of how certain decisions are made at each of these stages. In some teams, all referrals are made to the team and practitioners take most or all of their work from the team allocation meeting. These 'single entry teams' then vary in terms of whether the practitioner reports back to the team at later stages of the client's pathway, or whether the client is managed within a professional service pathway.

Table 1.1 shows ten stages in a client or patient pathway. This framework can be used to describe differences between teams in terms of how the team makes decisions about case acceptance and care management. Teams use this framework to clarify and agree decision-making for different types of clients or patients, and to improve their service quality (Øvretveit, 1993).

Table 1.1   A ten-stage pathway mapping framework for describing a team's decision-making

[Stage]				
1 Referral Sources	2 Reception	3 Acceptance for assessment	4 Allocation for assessment	5 Assessment
6 Acceptance for longer-term care	7 Allocation for longer-term care	8 Intervention and/or monitoring	9 Review	10 Closure

19

In the six common types of team process we consider below, we use fewer stages because the above detail is not necessary to distinguish the main different types of team process. Many teams have one general pathway for all clients. All clients receive an assessment, have a care plan, get a review and are closed to the team according to the same general procedure and decision-making process. Some teams have different pathways for certain clients, such as long-term or acute clients in mental health teams – they have different care programme pathways (Sayce, Craig and Boardman, 1991; Patmore and Weaver, 1991 and see Chapter 2).

Type 1: parallel pathway team

There are six common types. The first is the parallel-pathway team, which is how most network teams operate. Each profession has their own pathway, and team meetings are for cross-referrals, as in Figure 1.1 shown earlier. Chapter 3 shows a complicated example of a parallel pathway team in a community mental health team (Figure 3.1). In this team each profession had a separate pathway, as did the day-service team which was based at the same site as the team offices and interview rooms.

Type 2: allocation or 'post-box' teams

A second type of pathway is the 'postbox team' – named after the idea that the team meeting serves as a point where professional teams can pick up referrals to take back to the separate professional pathways. In this type of team (Figure 1.3) there are usually two pathways for clients to get to the team. In one the client is referred to a team secretary or a team leader, who then brings the referral to

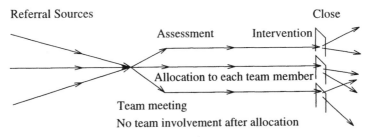

Figure 1.3 Pathways for allocation or post-box teams

a team meeting. In the other the team member takes the referral and brings it to the team meeting, if they do not decide to 'take the case' themselves. At the team meeting, team members take, or are allocated referrals by a team leader. Then each team member goes their separate way with 'their' client – they handle other stages without reference back to the team or to a team policy.

Type 3: reception-and-allocation team

This type of team is different from the second in that the team has a short-term response at the reception stage (see Figure 1.4). Team members take turns on a duty rota to staff the reception stage. In the fourth type of team pathway, the team has an assessment stage, before deciding whether to intervene and how to intervene:

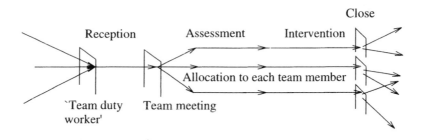

Figure 1.4   Pathways for reception-and-allocation teams

Type 4: reception-assessment-allocation teams

In this 'type 4' process (Figure 1.5), there are two allocation stages, one for assessment and one for longer-term intervention work. Clients are allocated first for an assessment which is more detailed than the one done at reception. This assessment is used to decide whether to allocate for longer-term work, and who should do this work. The team does not assume that the person doing the assessment will do longer-term work, if any is called-for, although for continuity it is better that it is the same person.

21

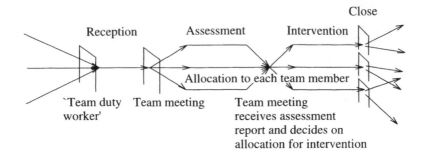

Figure 1.5   Pathways for reception-assessment-allocation teams

Type 5   reception-assessment-allocation-review teams

In this type of pathway (Figure 1.6) the team has a review stage, in addition to the stages of the Type 4 pathway team. At the review the team member working on the case presents a report to the team: they report their progress in carrying out the care plan and the client's current needs, and make recommendations to the team about any further work. Teams which are careful about managing their resources assume that team members have to justify 'keeping a case open' to the team – the team may be struggling to allocate other clients with greater needs. Some Type 5 teams also influence the decision by the practitioner to finish casework ('closure').

Justifying keeping the case open and review reports are ways of ensuring practitioner accountability to the team after intervention. They help the team to monitor client care, and to increase control

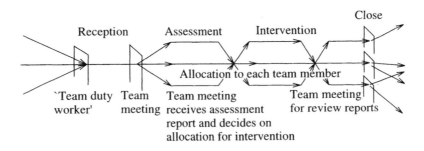

Figure 1.6   Pathways for reception-assessment-allocation-review teams

22

over team resources. It also calls for closer team integration, which requires a more bureaucratic structure and reduces team members' autonomy. In practice many teams are of the sixth type – a mixture.

Type 6:   hybrid-parallel-pathway teams

This approach to mapping client pathways helps to describe and differentiate teams (see Figure 1.7). It reveals ways in which teams can improve their decision-making and control resources more effectively. It also reveals the degree of case autonomy which practitioners have in different types of team (Øvretveit, 1986). Mapping client pathways lays a basis for using quality improvement methods which are more effective than the traditional quality assurance standards inspection approaches (Øvretveit, 1994).

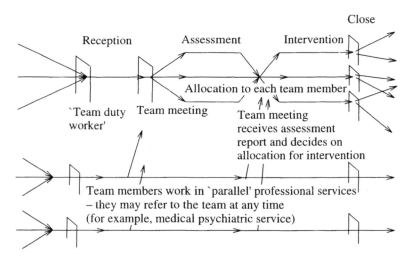

Figure 1.7   Pathways for hybrid teams

TEAM MANAGEMENT

The fourth way of describing a team is in terms of the management structure for members of the team. We will show the five main categories of team management structure shortly: general management; profession-management; joint-management; contracted-profession-managed; and hybrid-managed teams. First we look at some of the principles and issues which need to be considered in deciding or reviewing team management arrangements, in particular practitioner's autonomy. This helps readers to assess which of the five categories of structure is best for a particular team.

The purpose of professional practitioner management is 'to use resources in the most effective and efficient way to meet needs'. (Øvretveit, 1992). The aim of management is to get the best match between the most pressing needs and resources, over the short, medium and long term. Most traditional management is profession-management up to a certain level in a service management structure, above which general management takes over. In these structures, profession-heads have been responsible for assessing needs for the profession's services and allocating practitioners to areas of work to meet the most pressing needs. Lower down the profession-managed structure, operational profession-managers have directed staff, and sometimes decided how many hours staff spent on different activities or on particular clients.

In some professions, such as psychology and medicine, career-grade practitioners have a large degree of autonomy in deciding where and on what they spend their time ('practice autonomy' as well as 'case autonomy' (Øvretveit, 1992). Their head of profession sets broader parameters to their work than heads of other professions such as nursing and social work set for their staff. Therapy practitioners' autonomy lies somewhere in between (Øvretveit, 1992). In one sense all qualified professionals are self-managing: within the parameters set for them they match their time and skills to the needs and demands they face.

An important issue is what parameters are set to their practice and who sets these – the boundaries drawn around their work, within which they decide the best use of their time. Practitioners in a team may be over-managed: the procedures and directives may so prescribe their actions that they are not able to make even small decisions about how they use their time. More often practitioners are under-managed: the parameters are so broad that they spend their time and energy worrying about and establishing boundaries rather than deciding the best use of time within the boundaries. Team managers of many professions in a team have to recognise that the same procedure may result in over-managing some practitioners and under-managing others, even within the same profession.

24

There are thus two challenges in creating management structures for multidisciplinary teams. The first is establishing management which allows appropriate autonomy for practitioners from different professions and with different levels of seniority. The second is establishing responsibility for managing the total resources of the team: for assessing needs and ensuring that practitioners' time is allocated to where the needs are most pressing. Each profession and each practitioner have their own views on these issues. Team management is a controversial subject, raising issues of practitioner autonomy and control over their time, and of professions' self-image and status.

In fact many teams are poorly-managed. There is often no real responsibility for considering the collective multidisciplinary resources of the team and managing this resource in relation to needs, even in teams which are clearly set-up as services in their own right or as collective responsibility teams. Many profession-managers pay less attention to managing staff who are assigned to teams than to the staff they control directly, who provide profession-only services. Basic personnel management of staff in multidisciplinary teams is often neglected – no one pays attention to their professional development or standards of professional work. From the practitioner's point of view, the positive side of this is that they can gain a great degree of independence in their work, especially if it is in a community setting. This sometimes results in team practitioners developing interests which are not related to the most important needs of the clients served by the team, and there is no one in the team with the responsibility or authority to confront the issue. No one in the team wants to raise the issue because it appears that they are raising a personal issue which may cause bad feelings in the team. This is one of the many reasons why it is important to establish clear management structures for teams at the outset.

The practical starting point is to consider the management work which needs to be done to manage practitioners in teams. Although the details vary between professions and according to the level of seniority of the practitioner, someone has to be responsible for carrying out each of the following eight key management tasks:

- Drafting job description;
- Interviewing and appointing;
- Introducing the person to the job;
- Assigning work;

- Reviewing work (holding accountable);
- Annual performance appraisal and objectives-setting;
- Ensuring practice quality, training and professional development;
- Disciplinary action.

Traditionally, profession-managers have been responsible for each of these tasks, and we will see in the five models of team management structure below that profession-management is still an option for some types of team. Before we look at these models, we consider one aspect of practitioner management in more detail, not least because it shows the problems in creating a single approach to managing practitioners from many different professions. This is the question of supervision.

Practitioner supervision and professional politics

The subject of supervision is one of the most confused issues in team organisation and management. In my view this is because of the phenomenon of 'functional political interpretation' (FPI), where an ambiguous term or policy is interpreted by a profession in a way which protects or furthers the interests of the profession. This phenomenon occurs when a subject which is inherently complex and emotionally-charged then enters the arena of interprofessional debate and involves issues of professional control and autonomy. FPI is probably most marked in relation to the subjects of confidentiality and client access to records and quality, but let me explain how it arises in relation to supervision.

The initial confusion arises because the term is used within management to describe oversight and control of worker performance, and within professions to describe an educational and developmental activity undertaken in relation to casework. Within professions the managerial aspect is de-emphasised but still present. In the UK, with the advent of general management in the NHS in 1984, one of the arguments by professions against general management was the need for a more experienced professional to undertake supervision. General managers argued that supervision was central to their work and that they had the skills to do it. There was much unproductive debate because the different parties were using the same word to describe different things. Then social workers became a more prominent part of many teams, bringing with them a particular meaning to the term and different theories of supervision.

26

One result is that, in the 1990s, and especially in community mental health and learning disability teams, discussion of supervision arrangements first has to establish what each profession means, and then to clarify what arrangements within the team are required to ensure practitioners get the supervision they require. The following is one analysis which distinguishes between four different tasks and responsibilities. Supervision is a term used to describe one or more of the following:

1. *Task: clinical advice*
   A practitioner seeks out another, often more experienced, practitioner to discuss a client's problem, and to get their advice. The practitioner remains accountable and responsible for their decisions, and the advisor does not assume any responsibility for the case. An example is a therapist seeking supervision from another therapist. Teams can formally recognise certain practitioners with experience with different types of client problems, and with the skills to provide advice in a helpful way, as the people who can be approached by others to discuss cases. There is an acknowledgment that these advisors' workloads will be adjusted to take account of the amount of their advisory work.

2. *Task: clinical supervision*
   In this type of supervision a senior staff member has responsibilities for overseeing a practitioner's clinical decisions about client treatments, and is accountable for the practitioner's clinical work with one or more clients. They have authority to require regular reports, to direct and overrule the practitioner's clinical actions with the client, and to report to the practitioner's manager if there are any problems. Formal clinical supervision with this type of supervisor accountability is called for with newly-qualified or junior practitioners, to ensure safety, quality and for practitioner development.

3. *Task: management monitoring*
   Sometimes supervision is used to describe a person in a monitoring role who checks that a practitioner has followed administrative procedures, including those with a bearing on their clinical work, such as performing a care management role in the required ways. A person only undertaking monitoring will not be accountable for clinical decisions, and will not have authority to enquire into the details of clinical decisions or to direct these decisions.

27

4. *Task: full management*
Some supervisors are full managers, and supervision can mean full management where the manager is accountable for all aspects of the practitioner's work, including clinical decisions. For this they need the authority to appoint the practitioner, assign work, decide training, decide performance assessments, and to initiate deselection. If they feel that they do not have the expertise to judge clinical performance and to direct the clinical work of junior staff, they will delegate this work to someone who has or seek advice to do the work themselves, but they still remain accountable for the practitioner's clinical decisions. Often a full manager will monitor senior practitioners, and undertake both monitoring and clinical supervision for junior practitioners (for example a community nurse team leader).

In principle, all of the above four tasks could be done by someone who is not from the same profession as the practitioner who is being supervised (for example a psychologist providing clinical supervision of a nurse with the agreement of the supervisee's manager). Adequate supervision arrangements are especially important to improving quality and to supporting staff undertaking emotionally-demanding work. There is anecdotal evidence that the lack of such arrangements leads in time to lower quality, higher turnover and absenteeism and sickness.

Five team management structures

We saw above that there are a number of considerations in deciding management arrangements for practitioners in teams. Consultancy research has established that there are five broad types of management structure for teams (Øvretveit, 1993). The proposition in this chapter is that classifying a team in terms one of these five types can identify one of four ways to describe a particular team.

Type 1: Profession-managed Structure

In this structure (Figure 1.8), practitioners are managed by their profession-managers, each of whom undertakes the eight key personnel management tasks describe above, but each in a slightly different way because of differences between professions in practitioner's autonomy. This structure is most common in network teams, and can be represented thus:

Profession-managers

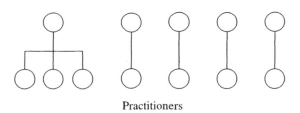

Practitioners

Figure 1.8   Profession-managed structure

Type 2:   Single-manager Structure

At the other extreme to the profession-managed structure is the
team where all practitioners are managed by one manager, who
undertakes all the eight personnel management tasks in relation to
each practitioner (Figure 1.9). This model is common in the USA,
Australia and in some European countries, but less common in the
UK, apart from in some community health locality teams. In some
variations of this model the team manager and practitioners may
have access to a senior profession-advisor to help the manager with
certain personnel tasks such as performance appraisal.

Team manager

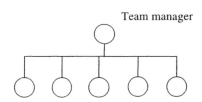

Team members from different professions,
fully managed by the team manager

Figure 1.9   Single-manager structure

Type 3:   Joint Management Structure

This structure (Figure 1.10) was the classic British compromise of
the 1980s, and especially popular in joint health and social service

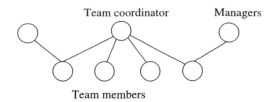

Team members

Figure 1.10   Joint management structure

teams. A team coordinator and a professional superior who might be inside the team agree who will do which of the eight management tasks.

Type 4: Team Manager-contracted Structure

In the nineteen nineties in the UK there has been a trend towards having a team manager with a budget, who contracts-in team members. Team members are often part of profession-managed services (for example a physiotherapy service), but are in the team under contract. This model (Figure 1.11) gives team managers control over team members through contracts, although the bureaucracy of contracts can approach that of the joint management agreements. It also allows team managers the flexibility to contract-in the skills that they need, especially when professions cannot recruit staff, and the opportunity to use private practitioners and others under short-term contracts. Profession managers retain the

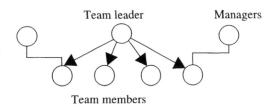

Team leader   Managers

Team members

Figure 1.11   Team manager-contracted structure

management of their staff, which can make it easier to recruit staff who prefer to work in a profession-managed service.

Type 5: Hybrid Management Structure

An increasing number of teams have a mixed management structure (Figure 1.12), with the team manager managing core staff, coordinating some under a joint management agreement, and contracting-in others.

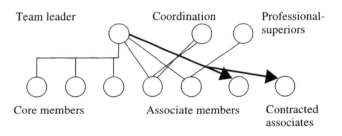

Team leader   Coordination   Professional-
                                                     superiors

Core members   Associate members   Contracted
                                               associates

Figure 1.12   Hybrid management structure

SUMMARY

This chapter has presented four ways to describe and distinguish a particular multidisciplinary team: in terms of degree of integration; membership; process and decision-making; and management structure. The ability to describe and distinguish a type of team is important for a number of purposes:

- To plan and design the best type of team for a particular population and service;
- To carry out research into which type is most effective, efficient or associated with certain phenomena such as staff turnover or client complaints;
- To enable teams to clarify how they are organised and the choices open to them for the future;
- To enable managers to understand and review teams for which they are responsible;

• To help staff applying to or just joining a team to understand what type of team they are joining and how it works.

There are of course other ways to describe teams (Belbin, 1981; Bion, 1961; Peck, 1985; Tuckman, 1965), and the above has concentrated on formal aspects of team organisation. However, readers will find that considering where a team lies on these four dimensions will help them to understand what type of team they are involved in, and to compare the team with other types. We will use these classifications in later chapters to consider interprofessional issues in each type of team.

References

Belbin, M. (1981) *Management Teams: Why they succeed or fail.* Oxford: Heinemann.

Bion, W. (1961) *Experiences in Groups.* London: Tavistock.

Hunter, D. and Wistow, G. (1989) *Accountability and Interprofessional Working for People with Mental Handicaps.* University of Leeds: Nuffield Institute.

Jones, R. V. H. (1992) Teamwork in primary health care: how much do we know about it? *Journal of Interprofessional Care,* 6, pp. 25–9.

Onyett, S., Heppleston, T. and Bushnell, N. (1994) A national survey of community mental health teams: 1 Team structure. Sainsbury Centre for Mental Health, 134 Borough High Street, London SE1 1LB.

Øvretveit, J. (1986), Organising Multidisciplinary Community Teams, BIOSS, Brunel University, Uxbridge.

Øvretveit, J. (1992) *Therapy Services: Organisation, Management and Autonomy.* London: Harwood Academic Press.

Øvretveit, J. (1993) *Coordinating Community Care: Multidisciplinary Teams and Care Management.* Milton Keynes: Open University Press.

Øvretveit, J. (1994) Why total quality management fails. *Health Services Journal,* 1 December, pp. 24–6.

Patmore, C. and Weaver, T. (1991) *Community Mental Health Teams: Lessons for Planners and Managers.* Good Practices in Mental Health, 380 Harrow Road, London, W9 2HU.

Peck, S. (1985) *The Different Drum.* New York: Bantam Books.

Sayce, L. Craig, T. and Boardman, A. (1991) The Development of Community Health Centres in the UK *Social Psychiatry Epidemiology*, 26, pp. 14–20.

Tuckman, B. (1965) Developmental sequence in small groups. *Psychological Bulletin*, 63 (6), pp. 384–99.

CHAPTER TWO

Planning and Managing Interprofessional Working and Teams

John Øvretveit

INTRODUCTION

The 1980s were a boom-time for teams in the Nordic countries, the UK and in New Zealand. But in the mid-1990s many working in health and social services began to question the cost-effectiveness of multidisciplinary teams. Service managers in both health and social services had to increase productivity and reduce costs. They looked more closely at the costs and results achieved by the different services they managed. Some felt that single-profession services such as a community nursing service were easily understood by referrers, purchasers and funders and easier to sell than a team service. Pressure on costs and competition led agencies to be more protective of their resources, and reluctant to assign staff to a team. Paradoxically, in some places the effects of reforms, rather than the intentions, was a pulling-back into agency- and profession-specific services and an increasing fragmentation of services. In others, purchasing agencies and joint health and social service commissioning groups continued to emphasise teamwork, but called for more information about activity, costs and effectiveness.

The reassessment of teamwork is long overdue. Many teams were created in the 1980s but many were fraught with problems and many of us suspected that they were more expensive and less effective than coordinated professional networks. More recently we have seen that the rhetoric of the primary health care team is no longer sustainable: GPs and others who actually have to create one have recognised that few actually exist, and that the few that did were not easy to establish. Many early teams were not planned and were badly set-up and managed. A few came through the problems and became effective working groups. But many remained mediocre and were more or less successful depending on the enthusiasm and energy of particular team leaders and core staff. In the UK and New Zealand we began to ask if care management was an alternative to teams.

As a consultant I get a biased view as I tend to work more with 'problem teams' and problems in interprofessional working. My biased view has not been altered by my other role as a researcher – there is little evidence of the cost-effectiveness of multidisciplinary teamwork in comparison to separate profession-services. However, it has to be said that there is not much evidence available and that research often does not distinguish different types of team. The good news is that many of the common problems in multidisciplinary teams are preventable. Many problems occur because managers do not set teams up properly and do not manage them once they are established. There is enough readily-accessible literature and experience about managing teams to avoid these problems. The main source of the problems, in my experience, is that no one group or individual is clearly responsible for and held accountable for setting up a team and for a team's subsequent performance. In the UK, New Zealand, and in the Nordic countries, the increasing interest by funders and purchasers in costs and effectiveness will rightly lead to more management attention being paid to teams and to interprofessional working.

This chapter gives a framework for planning and setting up teams which has proved helpful to planners and managers. It has also helped team leaders and team members to clarify the cause of certain problems in their team, and to understand that the problems are not due to any personal failings on their part. For readers working in or managing already-established teams, the issue is how to review and improve teamwork. The chapter describes how to conduct a review and considers the information needed for routine team management. The chapter also considers issues of change management in handling a shift in balance, or a radical transition, from profession services to a multidisciplinary service.

PLANNING A TEAM

The most important and the most difficult decision is whether to establish a coordinated profession team (CPT), or a collective responsibility team (CRT), as described in Chapter 1. There is no easy method for making this decision, but the decision is more difficult without some understanding of the needs of the population to be served, and of the existing resources available to the population. In this section we concentrate on feasible ways to assess needs for the purposes of planning a team, and introduce the idea of a team operational policy as a vehicle for setting up a CRT, and for some CPTs. We consider how detailed the initial team specifications should be in order to allow flexibility, but also to prevent predictable problems as well as that common phenomenon in interprofessional working, 'functional political interpretation' (see the end of Chapter 1).

How could friction in a team about unfair workload distribution between team members be caused by poor planning? In some teams one member or profession has many more clients and work than other members. Sometimes the team has information to show this, and the team leader takes action to keep a fair distribution. In other teams there may be no team leader or one with no clear role. Often there is no information or objective way of checking a team member's perception about workload. Over time, ill feelings surface as other team members make comments about overworked members always being late for, or missing, meetings.

Many teams are not planned on the basis of an assessment of needs of the population. Take one scenario: different professionals are assigned to a team by different profession-managers, as budgets or windfall-financing opportunities allow, and are expected to 'get on with it'. If there is a team base and more than average goodwill, those assigned to the team get together and agree a leader. Some team members bring their existing case load to the team, and new members start to take referrals to the team. In time it becomes clear that the mix of professions and the amount of each profession is not well-matched to the needs of clients being referred, or to people with needs who are not referred. For example, there is not enough social work or nursing time available to the team. Either other professions change what they do and 'role blurring' occurs, or the team starts a waiting list for some clients, and complains about insufficient staffing. Bad feelings can occur as some members of the team come under greater pressure and are always late for meetings or miss meetings to avoid feeling bad about not being able to take on more cases.

36

Team design in practice and in principle

This is not a caricature, but a description of how at least four teams I have worked with were formed. If the mix and amount of professions was decided on the basis of an assessment of the needs, then the workload imbalance would not be so acute. All too often the sequence of team formation is as follows:

- Problems in teamwork;
- Attention to team organisation;
- Agreeing team operational policy and procedure;
- Clarification of services the team should offer;
- Adjustment of team services in relation to other services provided in the area;
- Assessment of needs of the population;
- Readjustment of team staffing – mix and amount of professions.

The preferable and ideal approach to planning teams is the reverse: to start with an analysis of needs and finish up with the details of team organisation:

- Assessment of the needs of the population;
- Plan the range of separate services to meet the most pressing needs;
- Describe the role and purpose of the team as a key part of the range of services, and where the team base will be;
- Describe the range of sub-services to be offered by the team;
- Decide which professions and skills are required and the amount of each;
- Agree the details of how the team will be organised.

A team should be part of a 'system of care'

Note that the preferable planning sequence views the team as part of a range of services for a particular client group or population. For example, planning one or more community teams for people with learning disabilities or mental health problems should be done with a view to the part that these teams will play in a comprehensive

37

range of services for these clients. Although community teams of this type are often the first service established in an area, and have a key role in helping to plan and set up other services such as day services, the teams do need to be designed and formed as part of a pattern of services.

Similarly, primary health care teams need to be viewed as part of a pattern of services for different clients and health conditions, and in relation to other local welfare services. For example a primary health care team will need a certain staffing and organisational structure if the nearest hospital is some distance, school health services and local social services are poor, or other health services for ethnic populations are lacking, and the prospects for changes in these related services are low. The general point here is that, to plan a team, the team has to be viewed as part of a system of care. In some areas, care for certain conditions such as asthma or heart disease is being planned and organised across services and as a system of care. We have had less success in planning and organising combinations of services within a team in this way.

Why are not more teams set up in this more logical way, starting from an assessment of needs? One set of reasons is to do with problems with planning groups and implementation. In the case of primary care teams, it is often not clear who is responsible for planning and setting up the team. Responsibilities are often distributed across a number of managers, without anyone having clear coordinating responsibility. With other types of specialist teams there may be a care group planning team responsible for planning the range of services, which includes multidisciplinary practitioner teams, but the care group planning team may be ineffective. This often happens where there are frequent changes of membership, a wrong or too-large membership, or when the group works more as a forum for different agencies and professions to bid for resources, rather than as a corporate group with a realistic sense of the resources within which it must plan.

Even with a good plan there are usually problems in implementation. Finance is allocated through different channels and management budgets, and is not used for the purpose intended. There are delays and the financing situation changes, or managers committed to and knowledgeable about the original plan leave. One solution is for agencies to agree a project manager with responsibility for realising the plan, who makes regular reports back to the planning group or purchaser(s).

Needs categories and information

Another set of reasons for poor plans is problems in assessing needs, including difficulties in agreeing categories of need and in getting reliable information about needs. In acute health services there are two commonly-used categorisation systems: the international classification of diseases (ICD 9 and 10), and diagnostic resource groups (DRGs – numbering about 480 categories of diagnoses). Although these are not strictly-speaking systems for categorising need, they do give professions, planners and managers a common language to talk about needs. Thus those working with and in hospital services can measure and estimate demand and need for high volume conditions such as different types of heart disease, cancers, total hip joint replacement, and plan services for various diseases (Øvretveit, 1995).

We lack an agreed set of categories of need or of treatments for primary health care and community teams. Each profession and agency defines needs and treatments in primary care differently, as they do also in mental health, learning disabilities, child services, and services for the elderly. Our starting point should be the needs of people in the population for primary health care and community specialist services, but we must first agree how to categorise needs. This is also important for deciding team priorities and for deciding how to organise the team in a different way for different client needs.

The example of assessing mental health needs shows the problems and also some ways forward. The case example in Chapter 3 gives details of a needs assessment which was done as part of a team evaluation: here we note the primary categories of need which were considered. These were the number of people in the population of 90 000 who were estimated to fall into the following categories of mental health need: diagnosable schizophrenia, affective psychosis, depressive disorder, acute anxiety state, eating disorder, long-term mental illness, and 'other'. These categories are crude, not well-defined, and controversial, yet they were the best basis the team had for estimating and predicting demand and need, and for deciding skill-mix and other details of their organisation. Other ways of categorising needs we considered included:

- By a more extensive set of psychiatric diagnostic categories:
- By problem-based categories of mental health problems (for example 'low self-esteem', 'anxiety', 'over-stress');

- By types of service (for example a 'need' for a community psychiatric nursing service);
- By smaller geographic localities (for example electoral wards);
- By ethnic group, age, social class or sex.

One problem in gaining information about needs was that different services and professions use different types of mental health categories and definitions. The same category, such as 'depression', is defined in different ways by different professions and in different ways by practitioners in the same profession. If a service was to move to recording information about demand, as distinct from but related to needs, that all staff would need to agree a set of carefully-defined categories, which they could use after assessment to assign cases to categories. Doing so would also make it possible to monitor whether a team was meeting any priorities set in a contract.

In practice, planning groups and teams have to agree a set of five to ten major categories in order to plan and manage a team service, however crude these categories are. The debate about what these categories should be and their exact definition highlights the different views and philosophies of different agencies and professions. This is one reason why this work is often not done, or done by one profession or agency and their categories are imposed on the others.

The concept of a 'care programme' makes the task more manageable. A care programme is 'a service product or offering which is intended to meet the needs of a defined group of clients'. An example is a care programme for long-term severely mentally-ill clients, or for clients with profound and multiple disabilities. Two points about the concept need to be noted. First, a care programme is broader than a traditional needs category such as schizophrenia, hypertension or asthma. It encompasses a set of needs which one group of clients or patients commonly experience. At the broadest level 'services for people over 65' is a care programme because people over 65 are thought to have needs which are similar, and at the same time different, to the needs of people under 65. Because of the similarity of need and difference to the needs of other clients, it is often necessary to organise care differently for this particular group of clients. Having made this distinction, we can then consider possible sub-care programmes within this care programme, for example a care programme for people over 65 with organic mental illness. The second point is that the concept of care programme combines thinking about needs with thinking about services. .. compromise concept, part-way between a provider-concept such ‚ 'district nursing services' or 'vaccination services' and a pure needs concept such as 'difficulty walking upstairs'.

Thus, whilst professions and agencies may not be able to agree detailed categories of need, they can agree care programmes which are more specific than 'care for the people with mental health problems' or 'care for women and children'. With definitions of care programmes, planners can estimate need and teams can gather information about demand. This then gives a more informed basis for deciding team membership and deciding day-to-day work priorities within the team. I emphasise a more informed basis because information will always be inadequate, and lack of information can be used as a reason to do nothing.

An assessment of needs is not the only basis for deciding team membership and organisation. If we view the team as part of a system of care, or even if we take a purely pragmatic approach to planning, we need to recognise that there is a set of interdependent issues, each of which affects the other. These issues include: what other services are or will be available for the clients to be served by the team; which services should be centralised and which based locally; which work can generalist/primary care services do, and which should be done by specialist services; how will members be managed; and what is the purpose and work of the team? Because of the interrelation between these and other factors, it is important to start by being clear about what is fixed, decided, and will be relatively stable over the next few years.

FORMING A TEAM

In the information age we are becoming more familiar with the idea of a team without a base, where members do not physically meet. Indeed the concept of a 'virtual team' may well describe some health and social service teams, which are more a fiction of people's imagination that an effective working group. However, for providing health and social services, a base and close daily contact is necessary for most types of direct care teams, for a number of reasons. It is an absolute prerequisite for collective responsibility teams (CRTs), but some coordinated profession teams (CPTs) can function with only a set room for regular meetings (see Chapter 1).

...are many aspects to forming and developing close inter-...ional working in teams. In my experience not enough atten-...is paid to the two simplest and most important considerations: well-designed team base (for CRTs), and a starting operational policy framework. In the following we concentrate on how to draft an initial outline policy.

The operational policy as a development and management tool

The idea behind the operational policy as a vehicle for team development is that a management group decides the main features of teamwork. They agree and write a framework, which the team then uses as a basis for discussing and defining the details of how they operate as they gain more experience of working together (Figure 2.1).

I can predict with confidence that a team will not function as a collective responsibility team unless it has an initial operational policy which specifies the items described in the following. After looking at the list below we will consider how detailed the initial

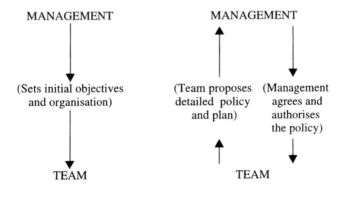

MANAGEMENT   MANAGEMENT

(Sets initial objectives   (Team proposes   (Management
and organisation)   detailed policy   agrees and
                              and plan)   authorises
                                                 the policy)

TEAM   TEAM

Team Formation   Team Review

● Team assess details of needs   ● Management and team agree
  and resources   details of organisation
● Team drafts detailed operational   ● Management and team agree
  policy   service priorities and plan.

Figure 2.1   Team operational policy as a framework for team development
and management

42

specifications should be under each heading because this ques
relates to issues of team flexibility and member autonomy. Opera
tional policies are also useful but not so essential for coordinated
profession teams such as some networks – in these teams each
member is governed by their professions' and agencies' policies and
priorities. In these teams an operational policy is useful to make
clear when and how the team members are governed by their
professional and agency service policies, and what flexibility is open
to them in relation to the team.

Team objectives and organisation should not be too-closely
defined at the outset. Higher management should require the team
to make a detailed report at a later team review (discussed below).
Once the team is working it begins to form a view of needs and
resources and can further define its operational policy. At the
review the team reports on local needs and resources, and proposes
the details of organisation which the team believe to be most
suitable for their work.

Operational policy headings

In drafting the framework policy, the management group needs to
consider and make decisions about the following. This list can serve
as a set of headings and checklist for the policy. Does your team
have written guidance about the following, and if not why not?

1. *Needs to be served by the team.* This has to go beyond a general
   statement such as 'people with a learning disability in the x
   area above the age of 18', or 'needs for primary health care
   services of those registered with y practice'. The initial policy
   should state categories of need or care programmes to give the
   team guidance as to the proportion of resources to allocate to
   different types of clients or client problems. For example,
   management cannot criticise a team for neglecting 'long-term
   severely mentally-ill clients' if the team is not given guidance
   about the proportion of the team's caseload which should fall
   into this category and some description of what the category
   means.
2. *Team purpose and work.* This section of the initial policy
   should make it clear whether the team is a network for
   coordinating separate professional services (CPT), or whether
   the team is a collective responsibility team (CRT). It should
   list any purposes other than direct client cure and care, such as

training and advice to other care staff and the proportion of team time to be spent on these purposes. Specific targets should be set for the team to achieve in a later section of the policy (item 13).

3. *Team catchment and boundaries.* This section describes the population the team is to serve and gives guidance about boundary interface with other services. The latter includes guidance about possible overlap, duplication and gaps at the boundary between the team's service and other services. Examples are clarification of responsibilities for care for people with mental health problems and learning disabilities, or primary health care team responsibilities for different mental health problems.

4. *Base(s).* The initial policy should make clear where team members and their offices, points of contact and records are to be based, and where clinics and other service bases are to be sited. There are often unnecessary delays in staff moving to a shared base, and these delays are not always the fault of management not finding a base but of practitioners not being clear that they are expected to move in and when.

5. *Team membership.* The number of staff from each profession, their grade, time allocated to the team, and any time spent in other teams and services. For each team member, a short paragraph on their role and the services they offer.

6. *Referrals to and access to the team.* Sources from whom the team accepts referrals, including whether the team accepts self-referrals. Whether any team member can accept referrals separately from the team meeting, either as part of another service (for example a stand-alone psychology service) or under agreement with the team. In further detailing the policy the team will describe how to make a referral and criteria to decide whether to refer.

7. *Team processes and decision-making.* This section of the policy gives guidance about procedures for managing work. The initial policy will only cover a few key areas, such as whether the team will have an emergency or crisis service, care plans, reviews, and when and why cases will be kept open longer than six months ('case closure'). Teams can use the client pathway mapping framework (Chapter 1) to develop their description of procedures and decision-making for different types of client.

8. *Care coordination* within the team and between the team and other services. The initial policy outlines whether there will be

a formal care coordinator role within the team for client being serviced by more than one team member. It will also give guidance as to how health teams will contribute to social service care management assessments, and how one full care manager will be agreed between agencies for certain clients receiving care from many agencies who need a single care manager.

9. *Team leader role*, responsibilities and authority. Of all the items to be specified in an initial policy this is the most important. Chapter 1 introduced different team leader roles in describing different team management structures. The role of team leader is discussed in detail in Øvretveit (1993, chapter 7).

10. *Supervision, professional advice and quality of professional practice.* This section of the policy gives initial guidance as to how practitioners will get access to advice to help them with complex cases, and about how the quality of practitioners' work will be improved.

11. *Case records and work recording.* Here management gives basic details of what type of case records will be kept. In integrated teams there should be one and only one case-file for each client, which should be held at the team base. It also describes access and confidentiality requirements. It should also define how records will be kept of referrals and workload, and whether two-week 'activity snapshots' will be conducted (see Øvretveit, 1985, 1986, 1991).

12. *Team management and reviews.* The initial policy should state which individual or group above the level of the team leader is responsible for the performance of the team as a whole. It should describe how and when team performance will be assessed.

13. *Team targets and milestones.* Achievement targets to be reached by the team set at six-monthly intervals.

14. *Other details* of operational policy, such as safety requirements, administration arrangements, holiday and sickness arrangements, etc.

Flexibility

The art in drawing up an initial policy is to specify the key elements, but leave enough open to the team to develop the details and to make the policy their own. So long as a full management review is scheduled, for example a year after forming the team, then management can afford to err on the general side if they are not sure of the situation which the team will find themselves in when the team becomes operational.

Two factors affect how flexibly the team responds to needs. The first is 'needs-related diversity': whether the team was structured with staff with the right skills and knowledge to meet the needs, and in the right amounts. Without appropriate needs-related diversity clients will not be served, will have to wait, or will get a service from a less-skilled member of staff. The second is the extent of 'task flexibility of staff' – the range of tasks which staff are capable and competent to undertake. Often there is intra-professional task flexibility, where one member of the profession can stand in for another. Collective responsibility teams have to develop inter-professional task flexibility – where people from one profession can do work traditionally done by another (one aspect of role-blurring or multi-skilling). This is because the broad structuring of professions in the team will never exactly match the demands put on it, and team members will have to mix and match.

This begs many questions as to how to achieve needs related diversity and staff task flexibility. It is not easy to overcome entrenched traditional professional attitudes and protectionism to achieve these things, especially when people are concerned about job cuts. There is also the danger that managers will not recognise some of the legitimate concerns of professions about competence, supervision and quality, which can get lost in what managers view as 'precious special pleading.' There is also the danger that the initial policy guidelines will be so specific about roles, tasks and procedures that team members will not be able to develop task flexibility.

Of course in coordinated profession teams there is less flexibility, as the team is made-up of separate profession-services with already-defined priorities and procedures. However, in collective responsibility teams the operational policy has to define roles and procedures in a way which allows staff the latitude collectively to decide which work and working relations are best for the priority needs. Yet it also has to be sufficiently precise to ensure that individual members do not pursue interests unrelated to the priority needs of the team, and sufficiently precise for others in the team to judge whether a team member is ignoring team policy.

There must be one individual or a group at a management level above the team, who is responsible for managing the team, and who is in turn accountable to top level management (or purchasers) for the team's performance. In between formal reviews this individual or group liaises with the team leader (for example the team coordinator, chairperson, or team manager). Sometimes the team management group includes profession-managers (for coordinated profession teams), or profession-advisors (for some collective responsibility teams).

In coordinated profession teams, the main management question is how well the meetings are working for coordination, communications and cross-referrals. In collective responsibility teams, management judges the team's performance in terms of how well the team has used its collective resources to meet the needs of the population it is serving.

The process of team accountability ensures that senior management receive a formal report from the team about progress and problems in order that those in authority can deal with difficulties which cannot be solved within the team. It enables management to redefine the place and purpose of the team within the wider service, and to check that staff management arrangements are adequate. For collective responsibility teams the reviews make it possible for the team to raise problems about over-control of members by professional superiors, at a level where negotiations with professional superiors can be carried out.

For collective responsibility teams these routine managerial reviews allow managers to make judgments about performance, to give the team feedback, and to negotiate future performance targets. The task of managers is to judge the team's impact on needs and consider with the team changes to priorities, services and organisation which the team should make. By doing this managers treat the team as a collective and reinforce the point that it is members' joint efforts and results that are important.

There are two types of feedback which teams need. 'Monitoring feedback' compares what team members have been doing with what was specified in the operational policy. To prepare for the review, management draws on a variety of sources of information about what the team is doing, including feedback from referrers, informal discussions with team members, and the team's formal report and statistics for the performance review. 'Evaluation feedback' is judging the impact of the team's service on the needs and demands of the population and is more difficult. It means asking whether the team's services and specifications are the right ones for meeting the priority needs. To do this managers need information about the impact and outcomes of the team's services on the population, and compare this with information about needs and demands. This information comes from referrers' and others' judgments, as well as from statistics on output and outcome. The next chapter gives more details in an example of how one team was reviewed.

Team information systems

Reviews always draw attention to the need to develop a team management information system in addition to, or instead of, profession-service information systems. Traditionally each profession-service separately collects and reports information about demand, waiting, work activities, caseloads, throughput (cases opened and closed), costs and sometimes outcome. Information in this form is not much use for reviewing or managing collective responsibility teams, even if professions are able to separate information relating to multidisciplinary team members from information relating to the stand-alone profession services. Indeed, it is often getting only professional-service information which precipitates management to question what type of teamwork is happening. Sometimes a collective responsibility team is operating, but changes have not been made to information systems to help the team move from profession-only to a multidisciplinary service. More often there is the rhetoric of an integrated team, but the reality of separate profession services.

A multidisciplinary work and client case information system takes time to create. Creating such an information system is not just a necessary support to full team working, and a way of stopping drift back into separate professional services, but is also an important way to build interprofessional working. Professions have to work together to design a multidisciplinary client case record system, agree access and disclosure policies, and agree common work categories and methods for recording and analysing workload. We learn more about other professions by working with them on these tasks than from special and often artificial 'getting to know you' training events.

Most professional practitioners hate forms and administration, even, or perhaps especially, social workers and nurses who have become so used to bureaucracy in their pre-multidisciplinary team settings. The general principle in developing a system is to create a good multidisciplinary client case record system, and abstract management information from this, rather than have two systems, one for client case records and one for administration and workload/activity information (Øvretveit, 1985, 1986, 1991). In the computer age there is no reason why a system cannot abstract anonymous information from each client case file or a team client master index/register for regular reports, without team members having to spend time recording and collating other information.

For collective responsibility teams there are two levels of management, each of which requires different information. At the level of the team, the management task is to get the best day-to-day match between the needs and demands faced by the team and the team resources – mostly practitioner's time and skills. In order collectively to manage team resources, team leaders and the team need information on the number of clients waiting and the severity and urgency of their needs. They also need information about each practitioner's caseload and the weighting of cases in order to ensure a fair work distribution and to recognise long-term mismatches between needs and skills in the team.

At the management level above the team, the task is to get the right mix and amount of skills for the needs the team is serving, and to define what the team should and should not be doing over the longer term, taking into consideration how the team fits in with other services. The task is also to check and take action to raise productivity, quality and reduce costs. For team performance reviews, the team should be reporting team information about:

- the volume of work, broken down by types of need/cases;
- quality, including process indicators of quality (for example waiting times, percentage of clients without a care plan, percentage of clients not reviewed at minimum required intervals, mand so on), and routine outcome measures (for example practitioner, referrer and client ratings of improvement at closure);
- costs, broken down by types of cases/key work categories.

From the management perspective, the minimum information required is to be able to show purchasers that the team is meeting contract, and to give prospective purchasers details of costs and quality. The system must be able to move towards costing and invoicing on a per-client or episode basis, and ultimately for an item of service, such as an assessment. Management information of the right kind, and which costs little to gather, gives a team a competitive advantage.

A checklist for reviewing a collective-responsibility team

The following gives a checklist of common problems for team leaders and managers to look out for in reviewing a collective responsibility team:

- Team meeting problems – frequent absences, avoiding issues, too many issues which do not need team discussion, unclear decision-making processes, inadequate chairing (especially allowing too much or too little time for different items).
- Emergency work driving out longer-term more effective work, or too much long-term work without review.
- Team members taking referrals or work separately from the team – under what conditions?
- Difficulty allocating new cases because members brought their old caseload to the team and never reviewed their caseload in the light of the team's priorities.
- No team influence over closure decisions, making it difficult to allocate new cases or work.
- No agreement over priorities, or priorities not defined in specific terms to monitor whether they are being met, or lack of common awareness of priorities and of ways of implementing priorities.
- No forum for in-depth case discussions of selected cases.
- Separate professional information and record systems, or difficulties getting information from others.
- Insufficient administration support, and inadequate team base (no good coffee/meeting area).
- Leadership with no authority.

SUMMARY

Most problems of interprofessional working in teams can be prevented by careful planning and management. Ideally a team needs to be planned by a group who are also planning a range of services, of which the team forms a part – a system of care. Agreement

50

between professions and agencies about categories of need is important as a basis for planning teams, and for teams to decide and manage their priorities. The concept of team care programmes helps to break down team service offerings into a manageable set of five to ten programmes. Programmes should be decided in terms of whether a group of clients exists with a set of needs which are relatively similar and different to those of other clients, and who may need different skills and care management approaches.

In setting up and managing a team, an operational policy has proved for many an essential tool. An initial policy drafted by managers should give guidance about key features of teamwork, but leave enough open for the team to work out the details, to make the policy their own and to respond flexibly to the needs and the situation which they find. Both coordinated profession teams and collective responsibility teams need to be reviewed by a manager or a management group responsible for the performance of the team.

The mistake which is often made is not having a formal review point where the team and higher management agree and sanction a detailed team policy. This is often because there is no structure and process for team accountability, as opposed to an individual member's or a profession's accountability – no clear management level and responsibility above the level of the team. Management reviews also accelerate the development of a team information system, based on client case records and giving work and costing information on a team basis rather than a profession-basis.

Planning and starting community teams: a checklist

The following lists some of the issues discussed above as a summary checklist. Decisions about one will affect decisions about others.

- *The context of the team's work*
  Do we have information about needs in the population, demands and current services?
  What services are missing, for which needs?
  What should be done locally and what centrally (managed or based centrally or locally)?
- *Type of team and its organisation*
  Whom is the team serving, which needs and what are the priorities?
  What is the purpose of the team? What difference is the team supposed to make, for whom, and what are the expected outcomes for clients of the team's service?

What type of team: coordinated profession or collective responsibility team? What type of pathway and management structure? What is the team catchment area and the boundaries with other services? What is the team membership? What type of team leadership role and what are the arrangements for team members' management?

- Details of teamwork
  What are the referral sources to the team, and can practitioners take referrals separately to the team?
  What is the main client/patient pathway in the team – is it described in a flowchart with key decision points noted?
  How are decisions made at critical points: responsibility and authority for acceptance, treatment decisions, review and closure?
  What are the arrangements to ensure care planning and coordination: responsibility and systems?
  What are the arrangements for case records, access and disclosure, and for collecting information about activity workload, costs and outcomes?
- Other
  Are the team's relations with other services described (for example overlap/gray area patients, continuity and communications)?
  How is the team managed and reviewed – who is accountable for team performance? What is the management structure and process for the team as a whole.
  What is the procedure for team monitoring, evaluation and reporting management information?

References

Øvretveit, J. (1985) *Client Access and Social Work Recording.* Birmingham: BASW Publications.

Øvretveit, J. (1986) *Improving Social Work Records and Practice.* Birmingham: BASW Publications.

Øvretveit, J. (1991) Records and access in Community Mental Health Teams. Service Development Unit, Denbigh Hospital, Clwyd, Wales.

Øvretveit, J. (1993) *Purchasing for Health*, Open University Press, Milton Keynes.

Øvretveit, J. (1995) *Coordinating Community Care*, Open University Press, Milton Keynes.

Evaluating Interprofessional Working – A Case Example of a Community Mental Health Team

John Øvretveit

INTRODUCTION

The community mental health team had been operating from their newly-built centre for 18 months. The team was not a disaster; in fact, compared to the previous lack of services, it was a quiet success and had many progressive aims. But there were problems or, as the manager put it, 'challenges'. The team management board decided to do a full review of the team on the team's second anniversary. Members of the board realised that they did not have sufficient information to do a review. They also wanted unbiased suggestions for improvements, especially concerning interprofessional working, and felt that the other teams which were being planned could learn from the experience of this team. Managers at a higher level in health and social services which jointly-funded the team agreed, and provided the finance for a short external study of the team conducted by the author.

The board stressed that they did not want a full evaluation but wanted information in a useable form to help with their review, as well as some ideas about how to make improvements, and as soon as possible. This chapter describes the short 'action evaluation' carried out by the author. The chapter illustrates through this case example some of the issues and concepts discussed in other chapters. It shows some of the problems which result from not building a team on the basis of an assessment of needs, but also how to introduce a needs and consumer perspective in reviewing a team so as to make mid-course adjustments once a team is established. It shows how difficult it is to establish interprofessional working, even in relatively ideal conditions, and how financing and competition in the UK is making it more difficult. It shows how, with the best of intentions, health and social services management can create an over-complex and over-controlling management structure which prevents rather than encourages interprofessional working and initiative.

But it is not all gloom – the chapter also shows ways forward which can help many other teams to do their own review and to decide how to improve different aspects of interprofessional working. It illustrates how to use the client pathway mapping framework describe in Chapter 1 to clarify decision-making and to measure multidisciplinary working – to show what actually happens rather than what people would like to think happens. It describes ten specific practical ways to improve multidisciplinary working which apply to most teams. It illustrates how to clarify the team management structure and to decide how to make improvements to team leadership to strengthen cooperation.

Structure of the chapter

The chapter starts with some background about community mental health teams. The example team we consider was a combination of day therapeutic services and different professional community services, all based in a new purpose-built centre. The team was financed by health and social services and had a team leader employed by the local authority social services department, and an assistant team leader employed by a health services Trust. Both reported to the five-member team management board, which included middle-level health and social service managers, two team 'user' representatives, and the director of the local mental health charity MIND.

The chapter outlines the action evaluation methodology used for the review, and describes the financial and competitive context for specialist community teams in the UK. Chapter 2 noted the importance of assessing needs in order to decide team composition and aspects of interprofessional working. This chapter will show one practical approach to assessing needs which was used for the team review. The information is limited, but better than nothing. The approach could be used by others with little time and resources, but who believe that some information about needs is necessary for developing teamwork. Later in the chapter when describing team staffing and workload, we will see that in the example team there are mismatches between needs and team resources. The final section then describes interprofessional working in the team and areas for improvement, and the chapter finishes by discussing the lessons for other teams and for interprofessional working in general.

BACKGROUND

Community mental health teams and centres in the UK

The original models for community mental health centres (CMHCs) in the UK came from the community mental health movement in the USA of the early 1970s. In the USA in the mid-1980s the emphasis turned to care management systems, in part because CMHCs were found not to provide sufficient services for people with severe and long-term mental health problems (Patmore and Weaver, 1991). Even though the evidence of the effectiveness of CMHCs in the USA was mixed, there was a rapid growth in CMHCs in the UK in the 1980s, doubling in number every year (Sayce, Craig and Boardman, 1991). One estimate is that the number of CMHCs in recent years increased threefold, from 81 in 1987, to 302 in 1993 (Onyett, Heppleston and Bushnell, 1994a, b).

It is important to distinguish between centres (CMHCs) and community mental health teams (CMHTs), especially for making comparisons. Teams (CMHTs) are ways of organising different disciplines providing services outside of hospitals. Some CMHTs do not have a common base, and may only meet weekly or monthly to allocate referrals. Other CMHTs do have a shared base, but may or may not see patients at the base. If the team base has facilities for seeing patients or running groups it is often called a CMHC or community mental health resource centre, but some CHMCs are full day-service programmes or day hospitals. A few CMHCs have drop-in facilities and a walk-in referral system. There is debate about how much CMHT services should be provided in, or even sited at, primary care settings (usually health centres or GP practices), as well as growing doubt about whether CMHCs are the best way to provide mental health services in the community, and a number of alternative models are being developed.

In this chapter CMHCs are defined as buildings, and CMHTs as ways of organising the work of different disciplines. It is common for a CMHC to be built and staffed to run a day programme (which may or may not have a drop-in), and for community practitioners to use the CMHC as their base, or as one of their bases. Often there is a day centre team and a team or network of community or peripatetic practitioners (for example, the CMHCs in Mold, and Colwyn Bay, Wales – Øvretveit, 1991). A common issue in such services is how much and what type of interprofessional working should occur between the day centre services and the other practitioners – should there be one centre team, or two or more teams, and how would or could a single large team operate?

Given the amount of resources invested in existing and future teams and CMHCs, it is surprising how little research there is on the subject. Most research does not distinguish between CMHCs and CMHTs. However, if we keep in mind the variety of types of team, then readers reviewing their team can make some useful comparisons between their team and findings about teams reported in a 1987–88 survey of 87 CMHCs (Sayce, Craig and Boardman, 1991; Patmore and Weaver's 1991 study of 12 CMHCs; and a 1993 national survey of 302 CMHTs, by Onyett, Heppleston and Bushnell, 1994a, b).

Action evaluation methodology

The aims of the action evaluation were threefold: to gather information to assist the board to review the team's operation, to make recommendations for improving multidisciplinary working, and to draw out the lessons for other community mental health services in the area as a result of the experience in setting up and running the team for 18 months. The author was contracted to spend 15 days on the study.

The methods used for the first aim were to collate the information which was available and present it in a form which the board, which included two users of the team service, could understand. The method for the second and third aim was to construct and refine descriptions of multidisciplinary working from interviews, centre documents and workshops with staff. In the course of this work the author was able to clarify with staff ways to improve interprofessional working, and to define future options for them and the board to consider. The study design aimed to involve the members of the team in reviewing their own practices and suggesting improvements. This method is a development of a collaborative action research method for short-term evaluation studies (Jaques, 1982; and described in Appendix 1 of Øvretveit, 1992). The main sources of information were existing policy and other documents, statistics and surveys, and interviews with centre staff, people using the service, and others outside of the centre such as GPs.

Three methods were used: the first was to collect and analyse the relevant documents, statistics and reports. The second was semi-structured interviews, which involved deciding whom to interview for the information that was required, and devising a semi-structured interview questionnaire. The interviews aimed to gather views and judgments about the questions listed above, as well as to give interviewees the opportunity to raise any issues which they felt important, especially concerning future improvements to the centre.

To investigate multidisciplinary (MD) working the method of 'client pathway mapping' was used (Øvretveit, 1993; and described in Chapter 1). This third method involves drawing client pathway diagrams which represent the stages which clients go through in passing to and through the centre. This methodology was chosen because, within the limitations of the resources for the study, it was the most cost-effective way of highlighting the outcomes for the client of the way in which the service was organised, and was easy for staff to use to analyse interprofessional working.

A framework for measuring interprofessional working and client participation was also devised. This involved staff and clients describing what happened and making judgments about the amount of interprofessional working and client participation which occurred and how it could be increased. Information for these models came from interviews with staff, cross checked by reference to client records.

Context: finance and competition in health and social service markets

Since 1991 in the UK, health-only CMHCs became financed in part or wholly from contracts which their parent Trust or units agreed with health authority purchasers. For other CMHCs which were jointly financed, like the example team of this chapter, finance came from contracts and from local authority grants and staff salaries. With many local authorities introducing a purchaser–provider split, following the 1993 community care reforms, the local authority financial element of a CMHC budget became less secure. Both health and local authority purchasers compare the value for money of CMHC services to that of other services. CMHCs increasingly have to compete for finance, and match or exceed other services' quality, flexibility, innovation and prices. Over time, not only will more of a team's services be purchased by more than one purchaser, but more purchasers will want to buy either a complete care episode for an individual client or a single item of service. In the UK, GPs and purchasing care-managers are setting the pace, wanting to buy services for one client, and often quite specific services such as an assessment or two therapy sessions. Teams have to be able to gather and provide detailed information and to quote prices quickly, clarify what they are prepared to offer, and be able to negotiate with an awareness of the issues for them and for purchasers. Team managers have to prepare teams for these changes, and to make sure that team members are aware of the changing market and the part that they play in winning, losing and keeping contracts.

The financial and competitive environment of the team in the study

The joint financing of the example team by the health Trust and social services meant that the team was to some extent isolated from the emerging competition for clients and finance which dominates the concerns of some other services. The team's day services were financed by the local authority, and by the Health Authority (HA) in the 'block' mental health contract which the health commission had with the Trust. Most of the community psychiatric nurses (CPNs) and outpatient services were also funded by this contract. In time the HA and the Trust will divide the block contract into different services, and the HA will contract for specific services. At the time of the review it was an open question as to whether the HA should contract for separate services (for example day services, CPN services, medical psychiatric services, and so on), or whether some or all of the team's health services would be contracted as a multidisciplinary service (for example a set price for an assessment or a particular treatment).

GP fundholders, with whom about 20 per cent of the people in the area were registered, contracted for CPN and outpatient services. They did not, in 1995, pay for drop-in or day programme services, which were paid for within the HA block contract. One consequence was that there was a financial disincentive for GP fundholders to refer to non-day services at the team. In addition, they would be expected to oppose any internal referrals from day services to other services without their authorisation. GPs will have an increasing influence over the health commission's purchasing decisions and their attitudes to interprofessional working will become more important. The health commission was planning to introduce devolved purchasing budgets for GPs (Øvretveit, 1994).

For their part the local authority paid for most of the running costs of the centre base and employed the centre manager and the senior day care officer in the day centre sub-team. The local authority also financed the social workers, their secretaries, the social service team leader, as well as the Borough social services mental health manager who was based at the centre. It was unclear how a purchaser–provider split was to be introduced into the local authority, but in 1995 the plan was that the social work team would be managed as part of a purchasing division in the larger adult services division, and would take on a fuller care management role. The consequences of the purchaser–provider division for the social worker's role and how they used their time was unclear, as was how the local authority would finance day services.

In summary, at the time of the review, few of the team's services were exposed to the scrutiny of purchasers, or were competing for patients and contracts. All knew that this would change in the next two years, especially if more GPs become fundholders or had a stronger influence over HA purchasing decisions, and if fund-holders acquired purchasing finance for day services.

The implications for interprofessional working were that staff and managers had to consider whether some or all of a team's services were best organised, 'packaged' and sold in contracts as a multidisciplinary service, or as separate profession and day services. For some teams, like the example team we consider here, the question is made more difficult by joint social and health financing, and by uncertainty about future arrangements for purchasing and provision in the local authority. The danger is that for some teams contracting and competition will drive a wedge between professions, and between them and day services, and undermine the cooperation which has been achieved. One option is a pooled health and social care purchasing budget, and a joint purchasing body contracting a team to provide an integrated specialist health and social service.

A PRACTICAL APPROACH TO ASSESSING POPULATION NEEDS AND DEMANDS

An understanding of the needs of people in an area is the starting point for a review of a team, for deciding improvements, as well as for effective team management and planning. A review must consider whether the relative proportion of resources allocated to different activities and services corresponds to the relative priority of different needs ('allocative efficiency'). Is there a disproportionate amount of resources allocated to responses for one type of mental health problem, and are other mental health problems or client groups, which are higher priority, allocated fewer resources?

In addition to considering amounts of resources allocated, a review has to consider response effectiveness: it may be that one response is very cost-effective and that a comparatively small amount of resources are required to meet needs. The practical question is thus: is the balance of resources between the types of mental health problems (for example client group or category) or between activities (for example interventions/treatments) right, given our knowledge of the needs of the area and of the effectiveness of responses? For example, if we know the number of people likely to be suffering from severe depression, and we know the effectiveness of treatments for this condition, then, from the total resources at our disposal, have we allocated the right proportion of resources relative to other types of needs and to intervention effectiveness?

In the case example the author had about three days to gather information about needs to help the board to do their review. The following shows some of the limitations of information in one area in the UK for designing multidisciplinary teams, as well as what can be done.

Measuring mental health needs

A measure of needs depends on how mental health and different categories of mental health problems are defined. Estimating needs for any service will always involve different views and judgments, as well as more objective epidemiological data. The following shows how different types of available data were used in the review to build an initial profile of needs in the area served by the team.

Categories of needs

The team served a population of approximately 92 000 in the northern half of a local authority borough, which had the same boundaries as the health authority (232 000 total population). We noted in Chapter 2 that one problem in gaining information about needs is that different services and professions use different types of mental health categories and definitions. The same category, such as 'depression', is defined in different ways. For teams to move to recording information about demand (as distinct from, but related to, needs), all staff would need to agree a set of carefully-defined categories, which they could use to assign cases to categories after assessment. Doing so would also make it possible to monitor whether the team was meeting any priorities set in a contract.

National averages

Using the categories of need and statistics from national averages, the normative needs of the team's population (92 000) are as follows (*not* controlling for population age, social class, sex or ethnic group composition):

- Between 180–450 people of the 92 000 population may have a diagnosis of schizophrenia (less than half (33–50 per cent) will be in contact with mental health services);
- Between 90–450 may experience affective psychosis;
- Between 1800–4500 may experience a depressive disorder;
- Between 1440–5400 may experience anxiety states.

(averages source: DoH (1993) *Mental Illness, Health of the Nation Key Area Handbook*

Area-adjusted normative needs

A more accurate picture for these categories of need could be produced by adjusting these figures to take into consideration the following characteristics of the population:

- *Unemployment rates.* On average, unemployed people have a higher rate of mental distress than employed people (one estimate is 2.5 times higher – source: North West Thames RHA survey 1990/1). The 1991 census for the borough shows a 7.3 per cent unemployment rate for men and 4 per cent rate for women

61

among 'economically active adults' (source: Health authority 1992 public health report).

- Sex: *women* may have higher rates of mental distress than *men* (one estimate is 2 times higher – source: RHA survey 1990/1).
- *Women bringing up children alone* have higher rates of mental distress than men (one estimate is 1.5 times higher – source: RHA survey 1990/1)
- *Social class*. In 1981 all the electoral wards in the area served by the team apart from two had less than 12.5 per cent social class (iv) and (v) composition (semi-skilled or unskilled). The other two had from 12.5 to 17.4 per cent social class (iv) and (v) composition (source: 1981 census).
- The proportion of the population from *ethnic minorities* is 12.4 per cent, and this includes: Indian (6.7%), Pakistani (0.9%), Bangladeshi (0.4%), Asian (1.1%) (Total: 9.1%); Black Caribbean (0.9%), Black African (0.4%), Black 'other' (0.4%) (total 1.7%); Chinese (0.5%) and 'Other' 1.1%. There is some evidence that some mental illnesses are higher in certain ethnic groups, although presented demand to statutory services is often lower.
- *Social deprivation* is associated with poor health and with a higher incidence of many mental health problems. One measure of social deprivation is the 'underprivileged area score' which is based on eight factors including socio-economic class, overcrowding, and number of very old and very young people. Most of the team's areas had a score of near the average, with two areas with little social deprivation.

It would have been possible to produce a more accurate picture of the amount of the four types of mental health needs by adjusting the national norms upwards or downwards according to each of the population characteristics listed above. For the purposes of the team review, the national norms were judged to be sufficient estimates for schizophrenia, affective psychosis, clinical depression and severe anxiety.

Local data about mental health needs

The 1991 Regional Health Survey found that the borough's residents scored higher than the average on a measure of mental distress, with a greater proportion of women, especially those bringing up children alone, also scoring highly. Nearly 50 per cent

of unemployed people received a high score for mental distre.
(source: HA 1992 public health report).

A community health council (CHC) survey of the quality of
primary care services for people with mental health problems
provided one direct source of information about needs. A questionnaire survey of one GP in each practice in the borough ($n = 57$)
asked, amongst other things, GPs to estimate the number of
patients within certain categories on the practice list. 25 GPs
reported 346 patients as 'seriously mentally ill' (SMI) a category
which covered schizophrenia, manic depression, depression or
personality disorder. On average this was seven per GP, but there
were wide variations. Adjusted for a 2000–per-GP patient list, the
estimates ranged from 1 to 23 people classified as SMI (other
research has showed an average of 10 per 2 000).

As regards the category 'neurotic illness' (covering anxiety/pho-
bias, depression, eating disorders, obsessive compulsive disorders),
11 out of the 25 GPs reported numbers of patients on this list that
ranged from 1 to 301 patients per 2 000. Nine out of the 25 GPs
reported no patients with obsessive-compulsive disorder, and three
reported no patients with eating disorder. The Community Health
Council researcher reported great variations in GP perceptions
about what constituted 'severe depression' (Miller, 1993).

Service demand

Information from existing services about the number of referrals
and about waiting lists and times may give some indication of the
needs in an area. This management information can be compared to
national norms to highlight areas for attention where there may be
under- or over-demand or under- or over-provision, compared to
averages. The national averages, adjusted for a 92 000 population of
the example team were as follows:

- 5 400–7 200 people are seen annually in general practice with
  diagnosed mental illness;
- 234 on CPN caseload at any one time;
- 1 800 seen annually by psychiatrists;
- 360–450 admitted to a psychiatric ward annually;
- 81–90 psychiatric inpatients at any one time.

(In a typical year out of 1000 people, up to 250 will consult their GP
for psychiatric problems, 17 will be referred to a consultant

st, and 6 are admitted to hospital or have consultant-led
e community).

ns – towards a needs-led team service

The available data thus suggested that, over one year, the team
should provide for an expected:

- 60–225 people referred who will have or be given a diagnosis of
  schizophrenia, and between 120–225 who will not normally be
  known to the service, but who will need outreach efforts to
  prevent problems;
- 90–450 experiencing affective psychosis;
- 1800–4500 experiencing a depressive disorder,
- 1440–5400 experiencing anxiety states.

The team also had a role in preventing the possible six suicides per
year, primarily through direct services to people with severe depression or through support services to GPs.

Although there was some information about some categories of
need, much information was not specific to the team's population,
and there were many categories for which there was no information,
especially for certain ethnic groups or electoral wards. The limitations to the information about needs is a handicap for all types of
teams. It also hampers service planning as well as operational
management decisions about how many resources to allocate to
different needs and activities. Collective responsibility teams are not
able to judge if they are using resources cost-effectively, or whether
moving resources from one activity to another would result in an
overall improvement in health.

A DESCRIPTION OF THE TEAM

In this section we turn to a description of the services provided by
the team, before looking in the next section at interprofessional
working within the team. The team's services based at the centre
included:

1. A drop-in programme (10 am to 2 pm, 5 days a week);
2. Day Activity and Group Programmes (5 days a week, on
   average 32 groups a week);

3. Social Work Services (SW);
4. Community Psychiatric Nursing Services (CPN);
5. Medical Psychiatric Out Patient Services;
6. Clinical Psychology Services;
7. Voluntary Services (MIND).

Services 1 and 2 were based and run entirely at the centre by the day staff, who were managed by the centre manager. Services 3 and 4 were based at the centre, with their own secretarial and office facilities and saw some clients there, but worked most of their time outside the centre, visiting clients' homes and GPs practices, as did services 5 and 6. The medical psychiatric service 5 conducted outpatient sessions using the interview rooms at the team centre, but did not have access to secretarial time at the centre. The clinical psychology service 6 operated in a similar way, but did not have secretarial support or space for records at the centre. One psychologist had a desk in the general SW and CPN open-plan office, as did the senior occupational therapist (OT). Voluntary service workers provided some services at the centre and had an office reserved for their use.

Staffing : comparison against national averages for CMHTs

A reliable comparison was not possible for the review because there was no information about national averages for day centre and community mental health team (CMHT) combinations. However, the following crude comparison (Table 3.1) provoked questions about skill-mix in the team, which had already been questioned as a result of the information about needs discussed above.

Processes

The team had three separate 'service processes' : the pathway of stages which a typical client usually passes through, from referral through to discharge or closure. These were:

1. the process for the drop-in service;
2. the process for the day programme of activities and groups;
3. the processes for the CPN, SW, psychiatric and clinical psychology services, which were broadly similar, but separate. Each profession had different arrangements for taking referrals,

doing assessments, planning and reviews; and different policies, for example about priorities and waiting times.

For the purposes of this chapter there is no need to describe the detail of these processes as we need to concentrate on aspects of interprofessional working. These processes are summarised in Figure 3.1, which was agreed by staff as an accurate representation, and which shows the team to have a 'type 1' pathway as described in Chapter 1.

Table 3.1   A comparison against national averages for CMHTs

Item	The Study Team	Average for 302 CMHTs (Onyett et al. (1994a,b)
Catchment Population	92 000	60 000
CPNs	10	3.83
Nurses other than CPNs (day 'sub-team')	3	1.22
Social workers	1 day, 4 field	1.87
Occupational Therapists (day 'sub-team')	2	0.95
Consultant psychiatrists	1	1.02
Doctors (other than consultants)	1	1.34
Clinical psychologists	1.5	0.9
Other specialist therapists	0.1	0.44
Administrative staff	4	1.87
Staff turnover per annum	4	1.6
% of caseload with 'severe *and* long-term mental health problems'	Information not available	57%

Although all described the team as a 'fully-integrated multi-disciplinary team', the pathway analysis showed clearly that the model was of separate services, sharing the same base: a 'coordinated profession team'. There were, however, cross-professional linkages forming, which we now consider in the next section.

INTERPROFESSIONAL WORKING IN THE TEAM

In some small teams, especially learning disability teams where staff share the same philosophy of care, cooperation often occurs naturally and systems evolve out of custom and practice. In larger

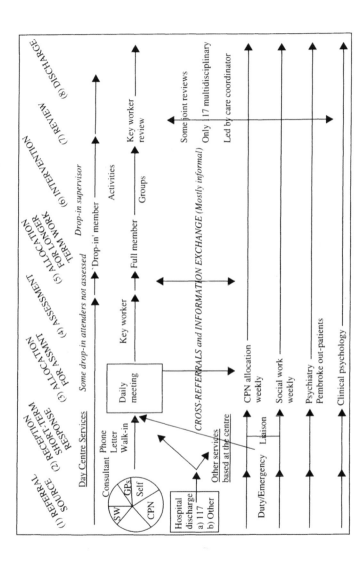

67

Figure 3.1 Client pathways in an example community mental health team, combining day and profession-services (a 'type 6-hybrid parallel pathway team')

teams like the one in this case example, where already working profession-teams are brought together at one base, action has to be taken to encourage and ensure cooperation – it cannot be assumed that it will happen naturally. Calling a group of people a team will not, of itself, mean that they will work as a team. Being under the same roof does not ensure that practitioners cooperate or even communicate when they need to. The same building is a necessary but not a sufficient condition for interprofessional working. The new purpose-built centre for the case study team made it easier, but organisation for interprofessional working also has to be built 'brick by brick'. As is usual, the details of organisation to ensure interprofessional working were neglected in the original arrangements for the centre. Social workers, CPNs and psychiatrists arrived and continued to work as they had always done, with some adjustments. Day centre staff were appointed and a day programme was created, with little involvement from other professions. Sharing offices was a big help and did lead to closer informal working. However, at the time of the review interprofessional working depended on 'corridor-contact' and on personalities, with the result that service coordination for clients or of policies was more a matter of chance than by design.

There is a tendency to assume that more interprofessional working is always a good thing. In some cases it is better for clients and can save time and increase efficiency. In other cases it can increase costs, for example by having too many meetings, and can result in a worse service, for example causing delays in decision-making because too many practitioners have to be involved. Often informal arrangements are the most cost-effective, but care has to be taken to create the right conditions to encourage informal collaboration.

One of the most cost-effective coordination mechanisms is a common coffee area with free coffee and biscuits always available, as in the example team. However, there is the risk that some staff may not cooperate when they need to: the larger the group the more formal the systems that are necessary to ensure cooperation, for example through the care programme approach for formal reviews. Attention has to be paid to formal systems, working through differences in philosophy, building mutual understanding and respect, as well as creating conditions for informal contact.

One method for deciding improvements is to assess where and when more (or less) interprofessional working is of benefit. This involves clarifying what is meant by interprofessional working, at the level of the individual client, at the level of management and policy decisions, and at the level of strategic planning. In the case example three methods were used as part of the developmental evaluation to describe the type and amount of interprofessional working and to consider improvements. The first was to use a framework of phases in a client's pathway through services as a basis for mapping typical pathways at present and for defining the work to be done in different phases (see Figure 3.1). The second method was for staff to use a more detailed framework to identify the specific type of multidisciplinary working in different phases. The third method was to invite staff to make suggestions for improvements using both of these frameworks, and in the light of their clarified understanding of the current arrangements.

Interprofessional working – conclusions

The conclusions to the review of interprofessional working in the 18-month old team were as follows:

Interprofessional working in relation to individual clients

- There was informal contact and exchange of information between CPNs, social workers and psychiatrists, in part because of working patterns which existed before the team started.
- CPNs and SWs on duty worked closely together (there was some pooling of referrals in the reception and short-term response stage (2)' of figure 3.1. However, the originally-planned multidisciplinary duty or crisis team had not begun.
- The day centre staff worked together closely as a sub-team, but the links between them and the other team services were largely informal, *ad hoc* and depended on personalities.
- Most SWs, CPNs, psychiatrists and psychologists wanted to know more from the day centre staff about how their clients were progressing in groups. Some took the trouble to ask or to seek out records to find out, and in these instances found the day centre staff very willing and interested in discussing their work and knowledge of a client.
- For their part, day centre staff wanted to know more from others about clients at the drop-in, or in groups. Sometimes clients were sent to the drop-in by CPNs, SWs or psychiatrists without informing day centre staff, and this had caused a problem with one seriously-ill client.

- Full multidisciplinary reviews for clients under section 117 of the Mental Health Care Act were reported to be effective, with all involved nearly always attending review meetings, and care coordinators did not report major problems in meeting their responsibilities,
- The problems arose for other clients for whom interprofessional working was necessary. For these clients the care programme approach did not appear to be working. Care coordinators and centre key workers reported difficulties in scheduling review meetings or in getting information from all involved. Often people do not attend review meetings.
- There was no care coordination for some clients who had contact with many day and other team staff. Some practitioners started work with the client with little understanding of what others had done, and were less effective as a result. Clients reported having to give the same information to different workers at the centre a number of times, some clients got contradictory advice, and there was a failure to create and carry out a mutually-reinforcing care programme.
- Some clients had many different reviews, which duplicated work (for example reviews by day centre staff, care coordinators, hostel staff, and others).

Interprofessional working other than for individual clients

Day centre programme
- Only two team members co-facilitated groups with day centre staff.
- The group programme was decided by day centre staff, and was reported by some other staff to be decided without consultation with them.
- Many team staff wanted to know more about which groups were run and by whom in order to decide whether to refer clients. They wanted to know more about what was offered, and how a decision was made about which groups were to be offered to a client and what would be done in groups.
- Many team staff were unclear about the process of assigning key workers and how the day centre services were organised.

Centre operational management
- The heads of profession meeting was described by many as a good start, but that there was no sense of corporate responsibility

for any aspect of the centre's operation. There was information exchange about management and policy issues and some alignment of policies, but each profession made their own decisions.

• The monthly multidisciplinary meeting for all staff was just for information exchange.

Centre strategic and business planning
• There was no interprofessional cooperation in strategic planning for the team or in planning for each service. Each professional service appeared to assume that their survival depended on planning and pursuing plans in isolation. There was little recognition that closer integration could strengthen everyone's commercial viability in an increasingly competitive market.

Options for improving multidisciplinary working

For more interprofessional working to happen in a team like the one in this case example, staff have to believe that the advantages to them and to clients are worth the efforts and problems of change. In addition, real and lasting trust, respect and understanding between professions comes more from positive experiences in cooperating in casework and day-to-day working than from team-building exercises and talking about cooperation.

In considering improvements, I started with four hypotheses about why there were not more arrangements to ensure interprofessional working:

1. The pressure of work at the time of setting up the team prevented too much attention to details of organisation for interprofessional working;
2. People were not sure which model or detailed arrangements would be best for a new type of service where there was little previous experience;
3. Each profession was afraid of losing autonomy and ambivalent about how much interprofessional working was necessary; and,
4. Practitioners under pressure of work and coping with a change of base were also reluctant to take on further changes to work practices when they moved to the centre.

Using the 'client pathway' framework, different staff identified areas where closer working would be of benefit to clients and/or reduce costs and delays. These areas are listed below because they are relevant to many other teams. The areas include: duty and emergency referrals; allocating non-emergency clients for assessment; assessment; allocating for longer-term intervention; one case file; multidisciplinary care plans; client reviews; groups; information exchange; cross-disciplinary training, consultation and formal supervision; and team influencing case closure. The options for each are summarised in Table 3.2, starting from the first stages of a client's pathway.

Discussion

In relation to multidisciplinary case reviews, option (6) below, Onyett *et al.* (1994b) found that only 0.3 per cent of the 302 CMHTs they surveyed did not have full meetings to formally discuss clinical work, and 62 per cent met as a full team once a week. In the review of the case example team it was felt that both clients and staff would benefit from multidisciplinary case discussions, but that clients would need to be carefully selected for detailed discussion as there was not sufficient time to do this for all clients.

The most sensitive area of interprofessional working was cross-discipline supervision, and this highlighted one barrier to increasing interprofessional working which exists in many settings. This is the concern which some staff have about future employment. For example, some CPNs believe that accepting supervision by other professions could put the value of their own senior clinical staff under question. In addition, lower-grade staff might be appointed if it was felt that they did not need to work unsupervised and that there was the possibility of supervision by other professions. In the case example team, fears were greater than necessary because of different understandings of what was meant by supervision (see Chapter 2). In all the professions there were underlying concerns about other professions encroaching into valued areas of work, and some had concerns about other professions' skills and standards.

One view in the example team was that it would be difficult to move to more interprofessional working involving some, or all, of the options below in addition to keeping the profession-specific processes. That is, to have some clients received and helped by separate professions, and some clients received and helped using the multidisciplinary arrangements for assessment and allocation. Another view was that it would be unwise to make a full and radical change to a full multidisciplinary process like an integrated team, although the specific reasons for not doing so were not made clear.

Table 3.2 Options for increased interprofessional working

Option	Advantages and benefits	Disadvantages and costs
(1) *A multidisciplinary 'duty team'* (eg possibly a 'crisis intervention' model) (a) for action on emergency referrals (b) for assessments	• Could create a single point of entry for all referrals and a single referral system (retaining the option for referrer to choose one discipline/ individual) • Spin-off effects from closer working between professions: eg greater understanding of roles and skills, understanding of when to refer to day services or groups	• May require a division of responsibilities within the duty team, with some having skills for specific types of emergency • May require training for some staff to handle emergency work • Requires changes to rotas and less time for current services
(2) *A weekly multidisciplinary allocation-for-assessment meeting* (All non-emergency referrals would be to a meeting for allocation for an assessment)	• Could ensure clients are matched to the best practitioner to do an assessment. Referrers are not always the best judges • Could be offered to referrers as an additional or experimental service, thus increasing choice and quality. Could still allow referrals to named individuals or services, as requested • Easier to arrange joint-assessments where this is thought necessary	• Unclear how many referrals can be delayed a few days for allocation at a weekly meeting. Some referrals may need a faster response than two to six days, or more problems could occur • Referrers may object to their referral being 'pooled' for 'matching', if their right to refer to a named profession/ practitioner is not retained • Different professions have different response times/ waiting lists. In practice, who has space to do a referral may decide rather than the best match of client to practitioner involved in this system

Table 3.2 (*cont.*)

(3) *A weekly multidisciplinary meeting for both:* (a) allocation for longer-term work, after an assessment. *(assessors make a report to the meeting, with suggestions for longer-term work if necessary. The meeting influences or decides what future work is to be done)* (b) agreement about who is to be Care Coordinator, if one is necessary	● After a specialist mental health assessment has been done, a multidisciplinary group can make better and faster decisions about the services which a person should get ● An assessment makes it possible to prioritise clients and needs, to ensure the most cost-effective use of resources ● A multidisciplinary group builds up a collective understanding of gaps in current services as a result of experience trying to arrange longer-term care for different clients	● Danger of too many multidisciplinary meetings, unless (2) and (3) can be done in one meeting ● Danger of unnecessary delays after assessment whilst waiting for allocation (eg two to six days)
(4) *One client–one case file* (a) Held in a team office (b) Held by care coordinator	● Ensures all records are together, so than any new workers can quickly get up to date with history and current involvement ● Helps to increase interprofessional working and understanding *(One survey found that 37% of teams had a single integrated record system (Onyett et al., 1994).*	● One worker who is intensively involved needs the file with them, or near them most of the time ● Could lead to separate duplicate record systems
(5) *Multidisciplinary care plans*	● Helps to ensure that each profession's work is coordinated ● Makes the care coordinator's task easier	● Some clients only have one or two workers involved

74

Table 3.2 (*cont.*)

(6) *Better systems for organising multidisciplinary reviews (eg one hour every month, with 'slots' for example for fifteen clients to be briefly reviewed)* • *for clients served by a number of practitioners* • *for one practitioner to invite advice and suggestions from a group about how to proceed with care for a client*	• Ensures that the clients most in need of coordinated care are considered by a multidisciplinary group • Staff are more likely to be able to attend one meeting scheduled at a regular time every month than many separate meetings at different times • Could reduce the number of duplicated reviews. • Lays the basis for a care programme system for selected clients	• Full reviews or in-depth case discussions would not be possible in one one-hour meeting every month • A client may need a review urgently
(7) *Co-facilitating groups*	• Opportunities for staff to learn from other staff who are more experienced in running groups • Spin-off effects in increasing cross-disciplinary understanding and respect • Clients benefit from a wider pool of skills and experience • Groups which cannot be offered at present could be made available	• Some clients may need urgent response whilst a practitioner is doing a group • Duty rotas would need changing • Practitioners are unclear whether it is more cost-effective to run groups or use the time for individual client work.
(8) *Cross-disciplinary training, consultation and clinical supervision*	• Clients get a higher quality service as a result of their worker being supervised by a more experienced clinician	• Some staff find it difficult to seek out or admit the need for help or training, and this can be even more difficult to do so from another profession

Table 3.2 (*cont.*)

	• Cost-effective use of all the skills and experience of staff for staff development	• More cost-effective for some senior staff to work through advising and supervising other staff
(9) *A multidisciplinary policy, or a team input into a decision to close a case (eg a decision to remove a client from the Care Programme Approach)*	• If a team cannot influence case closure decisions by practitioners through policy or directly, then it will be more difficult to allocate higher priority cases which are waiting • Closure decisions can be difficult for practitioners to make without guidance and support	• A multidisciplinary policy about, or direction to close, a case interferes with practitioner autonomy and responsibility, and could not overrule the practitioner's decision • Could be confusion between a team policy on closure and a profession's policy

An unaddressed issue was the question of closing casework, or active intervention, option (9). There was a view that cases should not be closed because 'preventative contact' was necessary to avoid problems. There is no doubt that in many types of team, some cases are long-term and staff have to be proactive to ensure contact and to prevent unnecessary readmissions, for example by ensuring regular medication. But is this necessary for all cases, and if only for some should this policy be applied to all? Unless cases are closed none can be opened, and in the example team some cases were being kept open which were of lower priority than those waiting. One reason why the issue was not raised by CPNs was that they had a policy of no waiting lists, and, in effect, this policy decided when and which cases were closed.

CONCLUSIONS

In the case example team, and in many others, there are few formal arrangements for interprofessional working in a number of areas where such working is known to be of benefit to clients and to reduce costs. The team's management structure was for separate day and profession services, each of which had separate policies and procedures which governed people's work. The day services and other services each decided their own priorities, training and other aspects of management, although there was some attempt to accommodate and adjust to each other's services. The team leader's meeting and the multidisciplinary meeting give two forums for exchanging information and for mutual adjustment, but there were no requirements to reach agreements. The commercial and other pressures were acting to reinforce profession-management and to undermine already weak cross-disciplinary links.

Apart from patients discharged to the team from the acute unit, there were no multidisciplinary assessments of the needs of clients referred to the team, and some clients would have benefited from such an assessment. There was no single multidisciplinary care plan for any of the team's clients, apart from certain '117 clients' where such a plan was required. All professions held separate files and care plans. The management review of the team agreed three ways to increase interprofessional working: meetings (for example client reviews), requirements and systems for information exchange (for example messages), and a common record systems (for example one client–one case file).

In the case example team, staff concerns about employment compounded the problems of separate management structures and policies, and were increasing the small amount of rivalry, suspicion, and work protectionism which did occur. Some staff had concerns about standards and skills in other professions, which was not based on an understanding of the facts and did not recognise others' skills and training. As a result of the team review, four of the nine options outlined above (2), (6), (8) and (9) were adopted, and there was some movement towards closer interprofessional working. Care coordination was improved by establishing regular meetings for reviewing a set number of clients on a multidisciplinary basis. An agreed care planning system, building on the existing care programme approach was also developed. However, these changes were in the absence of a higher level agreement about a future model of teamwork. The tacit agreement was to build stronger explicit cross-professional links, bit-by-bit, rather than move to a full collective responsibility team. It was clear, however, that the situation would have deteriorated without a formal review, and one or more professions would have withdrawn from the team. This example of interprofessional working serves to illustrate some of the general points made in other chapters, especially the importance of formal reviews for addressing issues which team members cannot resolve themselves.

References

Department of Health (DoH) (1993) *Mental Illness: Health of the Nation Key Area Handbook*, London: HMSO.

Health Authority (HA) (1992) *Public Health Report.* Hillingdon Health Authority.

Jaques, E. (1982) The method of social analysis in social change and social research. *Clinical Sociology Review*, 1, pp. 50–8.

Miller, P. (1993) A survey into the quality of primary health care services for people with mental health problems in Hillingdon. Uxbridge, Middx: Hillingdon Community Health Council.

North West Thames Regional Health Authority *Survey* 1990/1.

Onyett, S., Heppleston, J. and Bushnell, K. (1994a) A national survey of community mental health teams: 1 Team structure. Draft paper, Sainsbury Centre for Mental Health, 134 Borough High Street, London SE1 1LB.

Onyett, S., Heppleston, J. and Bushnell, K. (1994b) A national survey of community mental health teams: 2 Team processes. Draft paper, Sainsbury Centre for Mental Health, 134 Borough High Street, London SE1 1LB.

Øvretveit, J. (1991) Records and access in Community Mental Health Teams, Service Development Unit, Denbigh Hospital, Clwyd, Wales.

Øvretveit, J. (1992) *Therapy Services: Organisation, Management and Autonomy.* London: Harwood Academic Press.

Øvretveit, J. (1993) *Coordinating Community Care: Multidisciplinary Teams and Care Management.* Milton Keynes: Open University Press.

Øvretveit, J. (1994) *Purchasing for Health.* Milton Keynes: Open University Press.

Patmore, C. and Weaver, T. (1991) *Community Mental Health Terms: Lessons for Planners and Managers.* Good Practices in Mental Health, 380 Harrow Road, London, W9 2HU.

Sayce, L., Craig, T. and Boardman, A. (1991) The development of community health centres in the UK. *The Journal of Social Psychiatry and Psychiatric Epidemiology* 26, pp. 14–20.

CHAPTER FOUR

How Patient Power and Client Participation affects Relations between Professions

John Øvretveit

INTRODUCTION

'Patient' power', 'user direction', 'client participation' and other examples of the rise of consumerism in health and social services are not a passing fashion. Patients, clients and carers (in the following – 'people') expect to be fully informed about treatments and services, and to have a greater say in decisions previously made by professionals. Although many professionals pretend that these changes are not happening, some radical and some not so radical professionals have encouraged these changes in their work settings. However, there has been little consideration of how these changes may affect interprofessional working, or whether 'participation' is itself affected by closer interprofessional cooperation. Exceptions are discussions and reports by Steinberg (1992), Meyer (1993), and Briggs (1993).

How does increased patient and client power affect the way in which professions work together? Does it make interprofessional cooperation more or less difficult? Does it change the power relations between professions, as well as between professions and patients or clients? The sociology of professions has built up a body of knowledge about how professions relate to each other, and about changes in power relations between them. This chapter concentrates more on two practical questions for practitioners. The first is, 'how does increased patient power and client involvement affect the way practitioners work with other professions, inside or outside of a team?' The second is, 'how and when to increase patient and client participation, and should practitioners change the way they work with their professional colleagues to do so?' For the practitioner the subject is of interest because, considered separately, close interprofessional working and patient participation are both thought to be important in giving effective help to patients and clients with different types of needs. If this is true, is it also true that it is even more effective to combine close interprofessional working with greater patient participation? If so, how can we combine both in our service, and is it more difficult or easier to do both?

We will see that we can only give sensible and useful answers to these questions by looking at specific services and a particular person's needs: that the answer depends on what the person wants, on what we are aiming to achieve for them, and on how a service is organised. Many practitioners are alienated from the idea of increasing participation by dogmatic generalisations that do not apply to their clients or patients. Our route to answering these questions involves first defining what we mean by patient and client participation (the concepts). We then consider a framework for auditing participation which helps a service to describe the ways in which patients and clients are currently involved in decision-making. This gives us a basis for looking at ways of increasing this involvement where we and patients think there is benefit in doing so. It also helps us to understand how these changes affect the way we work with other professionals, and whether we have to first change our relationships with them before we can change the way we work with patients and clients.

The chapter concentrates on professional practice and service policies which increase patient and client involvement in decisions about their treatment and care. The aim of the chapter is to help the reader to:

- understand what is meant by 'patient power', 'client participation' and the many other terms within this subject area;
- reassess his or her own ideas about when and where greater or less patient/client involvement in decision-making would be of benefit, in a service you work in or are familiar with;
- assess the implications for how professions work together of changes in patient/client power and people's relations with individual practitioners;

• understand how patient/client participation is connected to the quality of service provided by a multidisciplinary team.

CLIENT/PATIENT PARTICIPATION – CONCEPTS AND PURPOSES

To introduce the subject we first note how the balance of power between patients or clients and practitioners has changed in recent years, and issues of language. We then consider four categories of types of participation.

Trends in patient/client power

There are two sources for the change in relations between patients/clients ('people') and health and social service practitioners, and between people and public welfare services. The first source of change is patients, carers and clients. People have been influenced by the rise of consumerism in the 1980s and expect more of health and social services. Disadvantaged and traditionally less-vocal citizens, such as people with a disability, people without a home, and people with mental health problems, have been influenced and helped by consumerism and rights-based movements and now demand a greater say in their own care and in what is provided for them. Politicians and governments have responded to this change in climate and sought to increase user power through reforms and approaches like the patient's and citizen's charter (DoH, 1991). For some politicians the motivation may have been more to reduce professional power than to increase citizens' power.

The second source is professions and disaffected professionals themselves. Many of us have found ourselves treating people in ways which we criticised in our training, and which are contrary to our values. The work situation we found ourselves in stopped us from spending sufficient time with people to make sure that they knew what was happening and to answer their questions. Some practitioners did not give in to the system but developed methods and philosophies, such as 'normalisation', which gave people more control of their care (Brown and Smith, 1992).

In the 1990s, other changes contributed to the increase in user power. Professional power derives from the professional's position in an organisation and from exclusive access to knowledge – both of which were affected by changes. Health and social service reforms,

81

in some instances, led to greater formal patient and client choice of service and of practitioner (DoH, 1990a). Practitioners recognised that their income or employment in part depended on attracting and keeping patients and clients. Purchasers and government bodies required services to offer more choice within the service, and to show that client and patient views had been taken into account. For UK specialist secondary health services there was a rise in 'referrer power' rather than patient power, especially where primary care physicians (GPs) held purchasing budgets for secondary care services. This also affected interprofessional working in some services. For example in learning disability and mental health services, community nurses, psychologists. therapists and others calculated whether their future was better as 'stand-alone' services, or as part of a team service which could be packaged and sold to GPs.

Patients and clients could also get authoritative information about services and treatments from sources other than practitioners – information which was often more easy to understand, but not necessarily more accurate. Newspapers published hospital performance figures; popular books, magazines, radio and television explained health problems and treatments; and booklets gave details of drugs and treatments (Øvretveit, 1996). Patients and patient groups became more knowledgeable than general practitioners about certain diseases, treatments and their prognosis.

These changes and more altered the balance of power between people and practitioners such as nurses, social workers, doctors and therapists. Along with these changes came a change in the language used to describe people seeking help or in need, which implied a different relationship between people and practitioners.

Language and attitudes

The words which professions use to describe the people they serve carry with them ideas about the relationship between the professional and the person, and about appropriate roles, behaviours and attitudes. Social workers call people they serve clients, users, recipients or beneficiaries. These words suggest a different relationship between the practitioner and the person to the words patient, customer or consumer. The words are important because they help to construct a relationship and they also assume certain behaviours and attitudes: the word signals to the practitioner and to the person how to act in a situation which is often uncertain and fraught.

Language is not neutral, especially in situations where people are not sure how they should be acting. The word patient is a familiar one, giving some comfort to people who know they are ill and who want help to overcome their illness. Being called a patient, and being given a diagnosis, can be a great relief when you do not feel well but are not sure what is wrong with you. What you are experiencing has a label, is recognised and real, and becoming a patient shows you that there is an accepted and possibly successful way to cope with what you are experiencing. The word connotes patience, and has its roots in the Latin word for endurance and suffering. These connotations fit with some professionals' preferences about how the people they serve should act; and they can help the professional if the person is patient, prepared to accept suffering without complaint, passively accepts what they are told to do, and does not expect too much.

Patient, customer or co-producer?

Some professionals who view the person primarily as a bio-physical object take the view that an active, questioning and challenging patient takes longer to deal with and is more difficult to help. It is often the same professional who winces at the words consumer or customer, which suggests the opposite of patient, and a transfer of power from the professional to the person in need of help. To them these terms describe their 'nightmare' patients – the ones who are not only difficult but who might complain, or worse. But their unease about the words has other sources. 'Consumer' conveys the idea of a person who takes in or uses an object, or consumes a service. A consumer may be passive or discriminating, but the term does not connote the idea of taking part in creating something. It fails to convey something important about the nature of health and social care – that the person and the practitioner(s) cooperate to produce the service – it is a 'co-service'. The term 'customer' similarly fails to convey the notion of two (or more) people working together. It carries with it the idea of 'the customer knows best' which is only partially true in health and social care. It is also misleading in that people do not purchase public health and social care services directly. And for some professionals it is dangerous because it emphasises the commercial economic value of the person rather than their human value.

Many of the commonly-used terms fail to describe or connote the kind of relationship which some practitioners seek to create.

'Patient' is too passive for many roles, especially in rehabilitation. It is too medical for many people with mental health problems and learning or physical disabilities. 'Consumer' and 'customer' are at the other end of the extreme, implying confidence, self-possession and certainty, rather than a willingness to form a partnership to work together. Whilst 'user' may be appropriate in some settings where the aim is to discourage any dependency, it gives the impression of someone exploiting the practitioner and the service and does not advance the idea of a partnership for co-service.

The point is not to add to the vocabulary of political correctness, but to note that these words are not neutral, and to put forward the idea of the practitioner and the person engaged in a joint activity. One way forward is to recognise that one term for all people seeking or in need of help is not appropriate for some people at some times. For example, the word patient may be entirely appropriate for someone about to undergo an emergency operation after a car accident, but not for someone in need of encouragement in rehabilitation after a stroke, or a person with a learning disability. The point is that we need to be more aware of the type of role, behaviours and decision-making which are appropriate for a particular person at a particular time in their care episode. Words like patient can sometimes make us less aware of the person's capability, needs and wishes and reinforce the wrong relationship and attitudes. In practice we will still use general terms to describe the people we are helping – we just need to agree on a term which is right for a particular service and setting. And therein lies one of the problems – can we agree a term with other professions? If not why not? Can one profession in a team raise the issue for serious discussion? Are they likely to be ridiculed for raising questions about the type of relationship team members should be establishing with people, and if so why?

The concept of 'co-service'

This discussion introduced ideas about types of relationships which may be more appropriate to some philosophies of treatment and to some settings. In these the practitioner and person work together in a relationship which is more equal than the traditional patient–practitioner relationship – a relationship of partnership, co-service, or participation. They do not 'deliver a service package' to a customer, but are engaged in an intimate relationship, where the person's own understanding of their needs and what they can do is critical – even when unconscious, on a trolley, going into an operating room. We are meaning-creating creatures. One of the things we can do is to help the people we serve to give meaning or a new meaning to their condition. The meanings we construct together may be significant to how the person perceives themselves and to the course of their illness or life path.

But how would these ideas affect the way in which professionals work with each other? Can one or two members of a team alone pursue these 'fancy ideas' and not affect the others' traditional practices? Are there any examples of teams which have created more participatory caring relationships, and are the relationships between practitioners in the team any different to those in other teams? First we need to look more closely at what we mean by participation, involvement and other terms. We need to be more specific about different type of person–practitioner relationships for meeting people's needs at different times.

WHAT DO WE MEAN? – TYPES OF PARTICIPATION AND INVOLVEMENT

Client involvement or participation can mean one of four things: giving the person information about what has been decided; consulting them; jointly deciding; or the person decides or does something themselves. Each of these are appropriate at different times for different people in different situations. Each of these can apply at the level of one person's care, at the level of service operations (for example informing people of a change in opening hours), or at the level of strategic planning (for example consulting people about a community care plan). In the following we concentrate on one person's care.

Giving information

Examples of involving a person by giving them information include explaining the side-effects of a drug, how to apply for financial benefits such as attendance allowance, or giving them written information. But we also give information in our body language and tone of voice, sometimes without knowing it. The message we give in these ways can be far stronger and even contradict our explicit message. The way we give information and our manner can be more, or less, involving. For a patient or client, a brisk manner, a

85

few words and a leaflet after waiting some time with many others in a waiting area is different to having an appointment, a calm setting, and time to ask questions of a practitioner who conveys that they want the person to understand the information and ask questions. Giving information can be worse than nothing if the person does not understand it, or the giver signals in different ways that they are only doing what they have to do. Communication is what a person understands, not necessarily the information we intend to give them.

When a person first comes to a service, the way they are given information is particularly important if they are beginning an episode of care or help. We often forget that people coming for the first time have little idea of what to expect, of what the service is like and of what will happen to them. Little things have a big impact, especially the first contact with someone representing the service. The way a person is first treated and the way in which they are given information signals to them how much they will be involved in what happens and how to act. It takes effort to later change the initial ideas that a person forms.

Giving more information, or giving it in a way which people can more easily understand and use is the least costly way of increasing participation. In your service, where would giving more or less information increase people's ability to make choices and decisions? Where and when are people information-hungry, and when are they over-loaded? Does your service give basic information about standards and rights and shape people's legitimate expectations?

Consulting

In this second category of involvement the practitioner still makes the decisions but is influenced by the person's views and wishes. When we 'consult' someone we seek their advice about what to do, but we decide what to consult about and what action to take. In 'consulting' the practitioner or the service decides when and how to consult, and how to respond to the person's views. There is the implication that if the practitioner or the service does not follow the person's views, then they have to explain why not, and show that they took these views into consideration.

The degree of involvement depends on how the person is consulted. 'Closed consultation' is where the practitioner or the service decides what range of subjects to seek people's views about – they 'set the agenda'. Most written approaches are closed consultations, although some have open-ended sections for any other comments. Services seeking to increase participation make assessments of when and where more consultation would increase a person's or group's ability to choose and decide, and assesses when and where patients are under- or over-consulted, sometimes by asking them. The audit framework described later in this chapter has been used for this purpose by one primary health care team (Øvretveit, 1991a), and by mental health and learning disability teams (Øvretveit, 1991b).

Jointly deciding (either has veto)

In one type of joint decision, either party has the right to veto a decision and to stop action. For example, for a surgical procedure both patient and practitioner have to agree, and either the patient or the practitioner may refuse to go ahead. More commonly, jointly deciding refers to a decision-making process, rather than the possibility of veto, although the possibility of veto can shape the process. It usually refers to the process and steps by which a person and practitioner consider a person's needs, their options and a course of action emerges. Many practitioners say that they make decisions jointly with patients or clients, and few say that they decide for them, but in practice is the decision truly joint with an equal say by both parties – would the patient or client say it was a joint decision?

In joint decision-making, power is shared and either can opt out or block the process. The inequality of knowledge between the patient/client and the practitioner is altered: the practitioner seeks to share their knowledge with the client so that the client can take a greater part in the decision about the best course of action, and sometimes about diagnosis and prognosis. The traditional inequality of authority is altered by the patient/client having access to other practitioners or channels for appealing or complaining against a decision. Some questions for services seeking to increase joint decision-making are: where would more or better joint decision-making be wanted? Could it be more effective or at lower cost? Where are patients prevented or over-encouraged from sharing decisions or actions?

The person decides

In many health settings, apart from emergencies and involuntary admissions, the patient makes the decision about whether to enter a service and about whether or not to undergo a treatment, at least in principle. For some decisions it is a legal requirement that the person makes a formal and recorded decision, as in giving a written consent to surgery. In the USA the attitude is that there is no such thing as minor surgery if it is your body. Such a decision must be an informed one, and the patient can sue if they can show it was not.

However, for many decisions about treatment or care people do not know that the decision rests with them, or do not feel that it does. People in the UK and Nordic countries do not always think of an appointment with a hospital consultant as a consultation, and of what the consultant says as advice. Practitioners do not often think of patients or clients as the decision-makers who are requesting the practitioner to pursue a course of action on their behalf, even though it may be a course of action suggested by the practitioner. As a crude generalisation, the more we move from acute emergency medicine towards non-medical community and social care, the more scope the person has to make the decision and to do things for themselves. Questions for services seeking to increase client or patient decision-making or self-care include: for which decisions would people want to have full decision-making powers, and would this be feasible, effective and at lower cost? Where are people prevented from, or over-encouraged to decide or do things for themselves? Can we give people sufficient help to make this decision or do it themselves? Would we be neglecting any responsibilities in giving powers to make such decisions to a client/patient?

Summary

By patient involvement and client participation in care we can mean one or more of four things: giving people information, consulting them, making decisions with them, or doing what they ask us to do or helping them to do it themselves. In thinking about participation in this way we have concentrated on who makes decisions and exercises responsibility – the person or the practitioner or both. This may be summarised in terms of a balance, where either the person or the practitioner makes the decision or carries the responsibility at any one time – shown in Figure 4.1 as a sharing of responsibility for a particular decision. In the right relationship, the person and practitioner together can share greater weights of responsibility than either could individually.

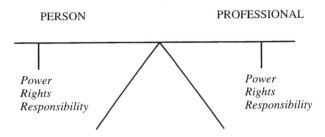

PERSON   PROFESSIONAL

Power   *Power*
Rights   *Rights*
Responsibility   *Responsibility*

Figure 4.1   Participation and involvement, viewed in terms of
responsibility and decision-making

HOW DO WE DO IT?

Even for small changes it is important to be clear about why there is
a need to change and what the benefits are likely to be. At a general
level, why should we increase participation? What are the problems?
And how should we do it?

Purpose and rationale for increased participation

There are at least five reasons for increasing participation. The first
is the therapeutic benefit. There is evidence that outcomes are better
for some treatments where patients have more information, a
greater sense of control and more involvement in decisions than
in traditional services (Morris, Goddard and Roger, 1989). For
example, one study found that inadequate communication about
drugs accounted for why 30–55 per cent of patients deviated from
prescriptions, and why 55 per cent of older people did not comply
with medications (DoH and HS, 1990). In mental health services,
different types of participation are therapeutic methods in themselves (for example group therapies, and user-run self-help groups).

The second reason for increasing participation is to organise the
service in a way which is more suited to people's preferences so that
they are more likely to use the service and it is more likely to be
effective. This is especially important for health promotion services,
for services with high non-attendance and drop-out rates, and for
treatments where patient compliance is a problem. A third reason is

that it sometimes saves money to increase participation. This has been shown in reduced length of stay and better outcomes when patients have education and information about their treatment. There is some evidence that for some procedures patients are more risk-averse and prefer 'watchful waiting', which results in fewer operations (Barry *et al.*, 1988). Getting patients and clients to do more for themselves can save costs, even if it takes more time to train and support them at first.

A fourth reason is to foster support and loyalty for a service. Taking trouble to get people involved in the service in different ways increases their sense of ownership. It reduces the chances of losing their custom and helps to get their support for service developments or to oppose closure. People who have been helped by a service, and who have given something back to the service by way of their time or money have a greater interest in the future of the service. A fifth reason is to reduce the gap between public and private services to stop the drift towards privatisation. Increasing patients' or clients' power reduces the differences between public and commercial services, and forces the public service to be more responsive.

Problems in increasing participation

Whatever the reasons for change, there are also many difficulties in increasing participation. In public services these often stem from the fact that practitioners and managers have to serve many patients or clients. It is often easier to ration time and resources in a service which takes a non-participatory or traditional approach. In these services it is easier to ensure that people who are less demanding or less vocal get sufficient attention. These clients or patients may get less time in a service with a participatory ideology – in such a service it is more difficult to hold this ideology and at the same time to set limits to the demands of those more vocal.

In some services it is questionable whether people want to be involved more, or whether they want more information. This may be because of the 'gratitude factor', a fear of reprisals, or learned passivity. In some services, clients or patients have difficulty expressing their views, or understanding enough in order to take a greater part in decisions. It takes time and effort for staff to learn ways to help them, and staff will not do this in services which are short-staffed or where there is no requirement or benefit for staff in taking this approach. Often there are no sanctions for failing to involve, consult or act on client views, or any incentives to do so. Not only is more time needed to take a more participatory approach, but it is also difficult to have a general approach for everyone – people differ in their abilities and desire to use information or make different decisions. What is welcome participation for one person, is purgatory for another. The main obstacles to a more participatory approach in many services are probably perceived as lack of time, lack of skills, and uncertainty about the benefits. In addition, there may be differences in view between professions about what changes to make, which may prevent one profession from increasing its participation.

Ways of increasing participation

There are different ways to increase a person's participation in their own care decisions and in how the service operates. At the level of care decisions, one of the most common and cost-effective methods is to give people written or verbal information about their condition or problem and about services. Another method is to have procedures and forms for involving the client in their assessment, for example by asking them to say or write down what outcomes they want from the intervention (Øvretveit, 1985, 1986, 1991). People can also keep and write in their case records, which can help when it comes to doing a review. Another method is to give practitioners training in sharing decision-making and to get them to propose when and how to increase involvement, perhaps using the involvement audit framework outlined below.

Some clients need help to define their own needs, to articulate their own views and to make decisions, and this help can sometimes be provided by advocates. Another method to increase participation is to help clients to form and run self-care and self-help groups. Ideally a service would find out from clients where they felt involvement could be better. Independent research into critical incidents – that is those situations where people felt they were well or poorly involved in their own care decisions – can make unexpected and useful discoveries.

At the level of service operation, involvement can be by consulting people through feedback methods such as focus groups, surveys and interviews. User groups or forums are less expensive but may not be representative (Øvretveit and Davis, 1988). This can also be a problem with user representatives in management meetings, unless there is an effective user-representation structure. People can also

91

play a role in monitoring and reviewing services, and in doing the review they can identify different opportunities for greater client involvement. Probably the least expensive of all methods is to invite a patient or a carer group or voluntary organisation to give suggestions about when and how to increase participation. This does raise expectations, and is not a good idea if a service is not genuine about making changes.

Voice:	extend areas over which clients can have influence (e.g. required consultation on community care plans, or hospital closure. Why not on appointment of staff?)
Choice:	increase service choices for a client, have competition, and give information in order that people can make meaningful choices. This will make services work out ways to be more responsive to what clients want. Increase choices when people are 'inside' the service.
Rights:	move from charters to penalties and legal rights to services, or to be consulted. 'Our customer promise – judge us against this'
Redress:	if something goes wrong, effective legal or independent investigation and response, if only to prevent the problem for others
Information:	make more information available in an accessible way.

Figure 4.2 Approaches to increasing participation

Participation and teams

In my experience some of the services which have done the most to inform, educate and share decision-making with the people they serve are multidisciplinary team services. One explanation may be that most of the team members share a belief in participatory practice and that this is associated with their general philosophy of care, such as 'normalisation'. In these instances there is likely to be disapproval of members who do not pursue this kind of practice, and support for individual members working to involve patients or clients. Support was found to be a critical factor in whether single-discipline social work teams carried through into practice their philosophy of participation (Øvretveit, 1986). This way of working was new, unfamiliar and difficult for social workers, and was only pursued in teams where there were systems and procedures that required client involvement in many different ways. In these teams, members not only discussed how to increase involvement in formal case assessment, planning and reviews, but dedicated time to learning from each other, to training, and to informal discussions about different ways to involve a client in the social work process.

HOW DOES PATIENT AND CLIENT POWER AFFECT INTERPROFESSIONAL WORKING?

In the following we consider two related sets of issues. First, how does the increase in patient and client power affect the way professions work with each other, regardless of whether practitioners are for or against the trend? Second, where one or more team members pursue participatory working in their own practice, how does this affect their working relations with other practitioners within and outside a network or team?

The effects of patient and client power depends on the particular decisions, types of patient/client and setting we are looking at. Increased patient power and participation will affect how GPs work with community nurses in a different way to how it affects the work of orthopaedic surgeons with therapists, or the work of social workers with nurses in the care of an elderly person returning home from hospital. It also depends on how closely practitioners work together. Increasing patient power in a rehabilitation service with a close-knit team may have a bigger impact on team members' relationships than on practitioners working in a wide referral network with little parallel working.

However, increasing patient power and client participation will affect relations between professions in most situations. The relationship between patients or clients and each practitioner has changed and will change further in the coming years. People can get, and some have, more information about their problem, about different services, and sometimes about individual practitioners or GP practices. In general people are less dependent on individual practitioners than they were even a few years ago, and practitioners are more concerned to respond to patients'/clients' wishes.

The patient/client–practitioner relationship is central to most professions. All professions seek to pre-structure the relationship in certain ways through national legislation and in their everyday practice. Creating the right relationship is critical to making a livelihood and to successfully helping a patient. Creating conditions to maximise trust are essential. Hence any changes in the nature of the relationship are threatening, something which we need to bear in mind when we consider the following changes.

Information about the service

In the UK, services have to give information about waiting times and about the range of sub-services which they offer. This is a government requirement and a commercial necessity in order to meet purchaser requirements. The need to do this highlights whether the service is a set of professional services, each with separate descriptions and waiting times, or an integrated service with a 'team' waiting time, or both. The need for an explicit written statement which publicises to people what the service offers makes different professions recognise what they offer collectively, and what they offer separately. It has made some professions reassess and clarify whether they are 'stand-alone' services or part of a team service, or both.

In some community teams this precipitated a move to closer cooperation and to defining an agreed multidisciplinary service. In some it led to increased competition and divisions between practitioners: in one service where community psychiatric nurses had low or no waiting times in comparison to psychologists, psychologists sought to emphasise their expertise, which was taken by some nurses as a devaluation of nursing skills. These changes in interprofessional working were as much a result of the market reforms and purchaser's requirements, as a result of increased patient or client power *per se*.

Information about condition/problem/prognosis

A second change which affects interprofessional working is that of practitioners seeking to be more open with clients about their condition or problem, either in response to patient or client demands or as a matter of policy. In general, patients or clients now seek more information about their diagnosis (or assessment) or prognosis than they used to, and are less prepared to accept uninformative explanations, or none at all. Patients are more likely to complain or sue if they feel they were not fully informed about a treatment or the options. This forces a practitioner to be clearer about what they do and do not know, and, whilst shaking the myth of professional omnipotence, it can also increase the person's trust in the practitioner.

The trend to more openness with people affects interprofessional relations in different ways. Ever since nurses and doctors worked together there has been the traditional difficulty of the nurse not knowing how much, or what, to tell the patient. In the past it was simple: the doctor made it clear what nurses could say, and, if in doubt, the nurse told the patient to ask the doctor. Where this remains the procedure there can be increasing strains on the nurse–doctor relationship, for two reasons. First patients put more pressure on nurses – they are more insistent and demand that the nurse tells them: Who knows when I may see the doctor again. Doctors have so little time and don't explain it well – you talk in words I can understand. Surely nurses have some idea, or are they not really knowledgeable about these things? The second reason is changes within nursing, particularly increasing autonomy, the concept of the nurse as patient advocate, and nurses' own beliefs and attitudes about what patients should be told.

One result is that a move by nurses towards greater openness can affect their profession's relations with other professions, and create conflict. Similar issues arise with professions other than nursing, especially in hospital and rehabilitation settings. With therapy professions, and some community nursing disciplines, two other situations are more common. The first is that the practitioner has made an independent assessment and prognosis, and shares this with the person. A problem arises when it differs from the one made by the doctor or other professionals. The person is confused and, where different treatments are indicated, does not know what to do. The second situation is where the practitioner has access to other professions' assessments and prognoses in the case record. The practitioner does not see why the patient should not know these, or inadvertently discloses an item which the other professional judged should not be disclosed at that time, or should be explained by them. This is similar to the traditional 'nurse dilemma' above.

Many of these situations, and the rise in patient power, point to one thing – the need for closer rather than less interprofessional cooperation, and for all professions to gain the same skills and knowledge to communicate effectively with patients or clients and carers. To be more open with patients, professions have to be more open with each other and work more closely together. Professions need to agree general policies about disclosure to patients, which are not just the views of one profession. Those working with each patient need to agree whether and when information is to be withheld from the person or their carers, and for what reason. Such general and individual policies are easier if professions carry out joint assessments, planning or reviews, especially if patients or clients are themselves involved.

A third change in patient or client-practitioner relationships which affects interprofessional working is the right of access of patients or clients to their case records (Access to Records Acts 1987, 1988, 1990). Many of the issues are similar to those noted above, in this instance concerned with whether one profession allows access to a record which holds information about the client given by other professions. Although a request by a patient or client for access to their record is rare, we note this situation here for two reasons. First considering whether, when and how a person has access to their record shows more clearly and in a physical way some of the issues noted above, where a person asks for a practitioner to give them information verbally. Second, a useful way of developing interprofessional working is for professions to discuss and agree a common policy about access and disclosure.

Increasing client choice and decision-making in care and treatment decisions

Involving patients or clients in decision-making can, like sharing information, bring professions into closer cooperation, or into conflict. The effects on interprofessional working of people taking more responsibility for decisions in their treatment or care depend on how closely professions work together, and which decisions we are concerned with. In loose-knit networks, where interprofessional working is mainly making referrals, the effect is less than in close-knit integrated teams. For example, in the UK, social workers in mental health or primary care networks have increased client and carer involvement in assessment, care planning, reviews and other decisions. Doing so has not had much impact on social workers' relations with doctors, nurses and others in the network. This is because practitioners in the network work relatively independently, and because clients feel that they can have a greater role in social work decisions than in more technical health care decisions: in general, increased participation in social work decisions has not led clients to expect the same in health care decisions.

However, where professions work more closely together in coordinated or integrated teams, it is more difficult for one profession to share decision-making with clients or patients without this affecting their relations with others in the team. If the client or patient is to be served by only one practitioner in the team (for example the type 1 post-box team described in Chapter 2), then team members can take different approaches to client involvement in decision-making. The issue then is whether the team should have a policy and procedures about patient/client involvement in different decisions which govern all members. Problems then can arise if different professions take a different view and cannot agree a common approach. The issues here are similar to those in agreeing a common client access and disclosure policy.

In developing multidisciplinary working, some teams decide to have a common assessment format which all members use to do an assessment (Øvretveit, 1991b). Agreeing the assessment procedure means agreeing how the patient or client will be involved in the assessment. This is even more important for teams which introduce joint assessments because the two or more practitioners doing the assessment need to take a similar approach with the patient or client. After the assessment in some teams another person may carry out the intervention, and again there is a need for consistency in the way in which the person is involved in decisions and this calls for a common approach or style within the team. Thus with closer-knit types of teams there is a greater need for a common agreed philosophy and procedures for patient or client involvement in decision-making. One way to increase client choice is to make it easy for clients to choose or switch their practitioner within a team or network. This too has implications for interprofessional relations, and can lead to resentment or competition if not organised carefully.

One of the effects of increased patient power and client participation is that it calls for better communications between professions. It highlights shortcomings in communications about a person's care, their assessment, treatment plans, and in updating any significant changes in their health status or social situation. These shortcomings are both a symptom and cause of poor interprofessional working. The causes are lack of time or an absence of an easy to use or automatic system for communications; distrust and lack of respect; fear of loss of power; fear of criticism or a practitioner's lack of confidence in their own abilities; and a belief that others will not understand what the practitioner is trying to communicate, or may misinterpret what they say or write.

Improving communications is at the same time improving interprofessional working. Some of the ways to do this include: a common record system (all have access to each other's files or one record file); getting the patient to hold or write the record; awareness-raising of what other people need to know, and why, and of the consequences of their not knowing; developing a common language and meanings; and methods for building trust.

AUDITING AND IMPROVING PATIENT/CLIENT INVOLVEMENT – A SYSTEMATIC APPROACH

Many services have not looked systematically at how they do or do not involve people in decision-making, and at opportunities for increasing people's involvement. Some services have made changes in an *ad hoc* way, sometimes because they have had to do so, sometimes because there was a general agreement that doing so was a good idea, for example giving patients an information sheet about their condition. A more systematic approach is to examine different parts of a care episode and describe how patients are involved at present and if this is adequate.

The ten-stage pathway framework in Chapter 1 (Table 1.1) gives a framework for auditing patient or client involvement. The framework can be used to identify the different opportunities at each stage for increasing involvement or decision-making. It is also a useful way to start a discussion between different professions about the subject and to identify areas of agreement and differences. In my experience it is more productive to have these discussions once a group has clarified the ways in which patients or clients are already involved in decisions. For agreeing changes to be made, it is better to discuss specific aspects of the care process and particular decisions, than to discuss participation and involvement in general.

Teams have used this framework to audit patient and carer participation in their service. To consider where more user influence and involvement would be of benefit, a team needs to ask:

- What are the key types of decisions in the care of an individual, in service operations and in planning future services?
- What are the decision-making processes and steps? Who is responsible and what is their authority and accountability?
- How do, or can, clients or patients influence each of these types of decision?
- What could, or do, clients, patients or carers do for themselves? What could we do to help them?

• What are the limits to increased influence or involvement? Where is it not helpful or not wanted?

SUMMARY AND CONCLUSIONS

People are becoming less passive in their contact with health and social care services, and they are also expecting more of practitioners. People's increasing expectations are to some extent in contradiction to their increasing power, if this power also means increased responsibility for their own care. The shift in balance of power from professionals to patients or clients has occurred at a time when professions are becoming more realistic about what they can achieve and about the significance of the person's part in their own care and treatment decisions.

People have more information about services, practitioners and treatments, and can often use this information to make choices and take a greater part in decisions traditionally made for them by professionals. People need information which they can understand in order to make choices and decisions. Practitioners have traditionally not been generous with the information they have given to people, often for good reasons. But information is power, and withholding it can serve to maintain power and dependency – in relation to patients and in relation to other professionals.

New terms have been used to describe the person seeking or in need of help – terms such as user, consumer or customer. These terms help to rethink practitioners' relationships with patients or clients, and the terms help to create new types of relationship which correspond to the changes in balance of power. However, terms such as consumer or customer can be as inadequate as terms such as patient for conveying the idea of an active participant in a 'co-service'.

Some of the changes in patient or client power have been welcomed and brought about by professions, and some have been resisted or opposed. Yet we have not sufficiently recognised how changes in the way practitioners relate to patients or clients are associated with changes in the way practitioners relate to each other. Changes in the balance of power between practitioners and patients or clients affect the balance of power between professions. These changes have an equalising effect and undermine traditional power relations. More equality between practitioners and patients or clients often means more equality between practitioners. It means that all professions have to acquire similar skills to improve their communications with patients and other professionals, and need to examine and agree common approaches to patient or client involvement, especially if they work in teams. In closing, two points need to be noted. The first is the danger of generalisation within this subject area. Some types of involvement and participation are wanted and helpful, and some are not wanted and harmful. For productive discussions between professions, and to advance research and theory in this field, we need to be specific about what we mean by participation and involvement in different settings for different people at different times. Some of this chapter has perhaps not been specific enough, but it has given concepts to help teams clarify what they mean by participation, and a framework for auditing specific arrangements.

The second point is that the increasing participation is as much a question of ideology and values as it is a question of evidence of the costs and benefits of participation. Even if increased participation cost more and was less effective, there would still be a moral argument for people assuming more responsibility and making more decisions that they currently do. However, having made this point we also need to note the lack of evidence about the costs and benefits of different types of participation in different settings, and the need for a more scientific approach in an area over-dominated by ideology. This involves looking for evidence for and against the propositions that increased participation is what people want and that it improves outcomes, and evidence of effects on interprofessional working. We need to turn some of the ideology into theoretical propositions for testing, and to consider the evidence for and against hypotheses such as:

- Patients always get better more quickly, and the outcome of interventions for clients is always more successful, when they are encouraged to make decisions which professionals would otherwise make about their treatment and care,
- Clients and patients have a greater role in decision-making when they are served by professional practitioners who work closely with each other than when they are served by practitioners who work less closely with each other,
- That better client or patient outcomes are achieved by services which exhibit high degrees both of interprofessional cooperation, and of client and patient involvement in decision-making,

- Increasing client and patient decision-making changes the relationship between professions. In multidisciplinary teams it changes the balance of power between professions.

References

Access to Personal Files Act 1987. London: HMSO.
Access to Medical Reports Act 1988. London: HMSO.
Access to Health Reports Act 1990. London: HMSO.
Barry, M.J., Mulley, A.G., Fowler, F.J. and Wennberg, J.E. (1988) Watchful waiting vs immediate transurethral resection for symptomatic prostatism: the importance of patient's preferences. *Journal of the American Medical Association*, 259, pp. 3010–17.
Briggs, S. (1993) User participation and interprofessional collaboration in community care. *Journal of Interprofessional Care* 7, (2) pp. 151–60.
Brown, H. and Smith, H. (1992) *Normalisation: A Reader for the 90's*. London: Routledge.
Department of Health (DoH) (1990a) *NHS and Community Care Act*. London: HMSO.
Department of Health (DoH) (1990b) *Caring for People: Policy Guidance*. London: HMSO.
Department of Health (DoH) (1991) *The Patient's Charter*. London: HMSO.
Department of Health and Human Services DoH & HS (1990) *Medication Regimens: Cause of Non-compliance*. Department of Health and Human Services, Washington, June 1990.
Meyer, J. (1993) Participation in care: a challenge for multidisciplinary teamwork. *Journal of Interprofessional Care*, 7(1) pp. 57–66.
Morris, J., Goddard, M. and Roger, D. (1989) The benefits of providing information to patients. Discussion Paper 58, Centre for Health Economics, University of York.
Øvretveit, J. (1985) *Client Access and Social Work Recording*. Birmingham: BASW Publications.
Øvretveit, J. (1986) *Improving Social Work Records and Practice*. Birmingham: BASW Publications.
Øvretveit, J. (1991a) *Primary Care Quality Through Teamwork*. Research Report, BIOSS, Brunel University, Uxbridge.

Øvretveit, J. (1991b) Records and access in Community Mental Health Teams. Service Development Unit, Denbigh Hospital, Clwyd, Wales.

Øvretveit, J. (1996) 'Informed choice? Patient access to health service quality information', *Health Policy*, Vol 36, pp. 75–93.

Øvretveit, J. and Davies, K. (1988) Client participation in mental handicap services. *Health Services Management*, August 1988.

Steinberg, D. (1992) Informed consent: consultation as a basis collaboration between disciplines and between professionals and their patients. *Journal of Interprofessional Care*, 6(1) pp. 57–66.

Preparation for Interprofessional Work: Trends in Education, Training and the Structure of Qualifications in the United Kingdom

Peter Mathias and Tony Thompson

INTRODUCTION

The purpose of this chapter is to examine the changes and trends in education in Britain and to identify the implications and opportunities they hold for interprofessional work and preparation for it.

The argument is that opportunities for interdisciplinary and interprofessional experience and learning could and should be consciously and deliberately built into the educational opportunities available to practitioners as they move along various pathways from school to work, to further and higher education and to professional training, practice and continuing professional development.

The interdisciplinary and interprofessional opportunities which can be provided may have modest ambitions such as an introduction to the perspectives of various disciplines and professions or highly ambitious ones such as the setting of new problems or the restructuring and reframing of established wisdom in knowledge or practice.

In setting the case for greater interprofessional and interdisciplinary opportunities and for the integration of various perspectives and approaches, it is assumed that professionals will rightly continue to strive for differentiation, specialisation and the development of profession-specific as well as common knowledge and skills. These are not therefore arguments for general, generic approaches to education and training which fail to recognise the plurality, diversity and specialisation of the professions active in health and social care. They are arguments for the creation of new opportunities for understanding and for the prevention of the fragmentation and separation between professions which can so easily damage people who use the health and social services.

The chapter will consider:

1. The range of professions involved in the care sector;
2. Trends and changes in education;
3. General National Vocational Qualifications and National Vocational Qualifications (in Scotland General Scottish Vocational Qualifications and Scottish Vocational Qualifications);
4. The use of credits and modules and further and higher education.

THE PROFESSIONS

The range of professions which contribute to health and social care is very wide and the number of organisations which have an interest in professional training programmes and the range of skills available to the services wider still. At a conference held in London in 1993 to discuss professional and occupational standards in the care sector there were representatives of 34 organisations (see Table 5.1). It is clear from the conference report that the different organisations had varying interests in relation to:

- the development of standards;
- the use of standards in the development and specification of qualifications;
- the creation of systems to award qualifications and assure their quality as national awards;
- the use of standards and qualifications as part of the requirement for registration with a professional association or statutory regulatory body;
- the establishment of educational and training programmes to prepare practitioners to work to the standards

(JAB, 1993)

Table 5.1   Organisations taking part in a conference in January 1993 on professional and occupational standards in the care sector

---

British Association of Social Work
British Dietetic Association
British Psychological Society
British Red Cross
Business and Technology Education Council (BTEC)
Care Sector Consortium (now the Occupational Standards Council for Health and Social Care)
Central Council for Education and Training in Social Work
Chartered Society of Physiotherapy
City and Guilds
College of Occupational Therapists
College of Radiographers
College of Speech and Language Therapists
Council for Professions Supplementary to Medicine
Criminal Justice Sector
Dental Laboratories Association
Examinations Board for Dental Hygienists
Federation of Community Work Training Groups
General Dental Council
General Medical Council
Health Education Authority
Local Government Management Board
National Health Management Executives
Open University
National Care Homes Association
Registered Nursing Home Association
Royal College of Nursing
Royal Institute of Public Health and Hygiene
Scottish Vocational and Education Council
St John Ambulance
Social Care Association
Society of Chiropodists
United Kingdom Central Council for Nursing, Midwifery and Health Visiting
English National Board for Nursing, Midwifery and Health Visiting
Welsh Common Health Services Authority
Four other organisations sent apologies

Source: Joint Awarding Bodies (JAB), 1993

Some of the organisations present specialised in one or another of the above activities, or were bound by statutes or constitutions which limited the range of their interest. However, professional associations tended to have interests across many of the activities

105

amongst which the effectiveness of education and training and control over the content of programmes of professional training were considered to be extremely important. Even if not directly responsible for them, the majority of the organisations were interested in professional and occupational standards, in how best to equip practitioners to contribute to services which are changing rapidly, and in how best to take advantage of changes in educational thinking and practice. Changes and trends in education are therefore relevant to both intra- and inter-professional debate.

CHANGES AND TRENDS IN EDUCATION IN BRITAIN

'Government policy for education and training focuses on the aims of:

(a) promoting parity of esteem between academic and vocational qualifications;
(b) engendering a culture of lifetime learning in both organisations and individuals;
(c) increasing participation in higher education.'
(Clifton, Thompson and Brown, 1994)

Clifton, Thompson and Brown review the literature and trends in education and training in offering their report 'Training and Education in Transition: Bridging Vocational and Academic Models in an Interdisciplinary Perspective' as a guide for those who are responsible for organising, planning or purchasing training and education in the health and social services. They argue that in the conditions which applied in Britain in 1994: 'The methodology of (a) defining employment needs (based on service user needs) leading to (b) an assessment of staff development needs, which generates (c) the learning outcomes and competences which training and education are required to deliver . . . can be seen as an approach which will allow bridging between academic, vocational and interdisciplinary training and education.'

Reform of the educational system and the introduction of a comprehensive framework of occupational qualifications alongside the academic has been a high priority in the UK marked by the establishment of the National Council for Vocational Qualifications

(NCVQ) and its subsequent work with SCOTVEC (the Scottish Vocational Education Council).

The National Council for Vocational Qualifications (NCVQ) portrays the relationship between the various vocational and academic qualifications available in Britain in the following way:

A national qualifications framework

The framework of qualifications in Britain is usually referred to as having three routes or pathways, one academic (GCSE, A-level) and two vocational (GNVQ, NVQ). However, the distinction between the academic and vocational is not really very helpful or very accurate. For example, Dearing (1996) in the government sponsored 'Review of Qualifications for 16–19 year olds' argues that consideration should be given to the creation of a common family of National Certificates within which there might be an award which recognises achievement in advanced level work, whether through vocational or academic qualifications or a combination of both. The Dearing Report also suggests that the merger of the Department for Education with the Employment Department might be followed by joint work and possibly merger of the NCVQ with the Schools Curriculum Assessment Authority (SCAA). The report argues that the rigour and cost-effectiveness of assessment should be examined and that the qualifications framework should reflect the idea of life-long learning and should recognise that people will learn in a variety of ways through work or education institutions or a combination of both.

Whilst the Dearing review is primarily concerned with qualifications for 16–19 year olds many of the points it makes apply to higher education and qualifications for older people, where choice and flexibility coupled with rigour and integrity are equally important.

Higher education

The Higher Education Quality Council (HEQC, 1994), for example, makes over 100 recommendations in a report of a project about access, choice and mobility in higher education.

One of the key recommendations of the HEQC report which is called 'Choosing to Change' is No. 30.

'We recommend that HEQC (Higher Education Quality Council), NCVQ, FEU (Further Education Unit) and the representative bodies of institutions in higher and further education actively promote the specifications of the single unified credit framework and assist institutions and others to adjust to the arrangements over time. Moreover, we recommend that professional bodies and employers be consulted to explain the proposed arrangements and that the HEQC assists this consultation process by publishing in consultation with ECCTIS (Educational Counselling and Credit Transfer Information Service) a draft list of parallel credit ratings for professional body programmes and accredited company training.'
(p. 167)

These reports, with their language of credits, units of competence, links and ladders between the vocational and academic, between educational institutes, employers and professional bodies foresee a time when: (i) learning, however it takes place, will somehow be credited within national qualification structures; (ii) people will invest in their own learning and professional development which will continue throughout their working life; and (iii) parts of the qualification structure will be based directly on occupational standards agreed by employment interests. Coats and Mitchell describe this latter approach in more detail when discussing the Functional Map of Health and Social Care in Chapter 8 of this book.

The implications of these reforms and changes in thinking about the vocational, the academic and the nature of qualifications for interprofessional learning are at least two-fold:

1. General education, given a vocational twist through GNVQs and NVQs, may impart a basic cross-professional, whole-industry perspective to the thinking of practitioners of the future because interdisciplinary, interprofessional work will be embedded in educational experience which will be informed by the needs of employers in the health and social services;
2. Credit frameworks and modular structures, whether competence or learning-outcome based, will allow practitioners in training at various levels the opportunities to move across modules based on various disciplines constrained only by the range of their own interests, the guidance and control of regulatory bodies and the policies of funding agencies.

GENERAL NATIONAL VOCATIONAL QUALIFICATIONS AND NATIONAL VOCATIONAL QUALIFICATIONS

Many aspects of general education such as GCSE and A-levels will be familiar to most readers but the GNVQ approach may not be, and it will be described in some detail in order to illustrate the argument that a decidedly vocational approach can lead to greater interprofessional and interdisciplinary perspectives within qualifications.

GNVQs in Health and Social Care draw on ideas and practices in the fields of health and social care, and intend to equip students to progress towards higher/further education or into work. GNVQs exist at the Foundation, Intermediate and Advanced levels shown previously in Figure 5.1. In contrast to NVQs which are competence-based requiring demonstration of performance in paid or unpaid work, GNVQs define learning outcomes and educational objectives.

Students wishing to move into training programmes preparing for entry into the health and social care professions may take a number of GNVQ routes but will probably be attracted to GNVQs in Health and Social Care or, if they are wishing to enter one of the science-based professions, the GNVQ in Science.

GNVQs are divided into units and at each level of the framework they consist of mandatory, optional and additional units. The mandatory units are produced and set by the National Council for Vocational Qualifications. The optional and additional units are produced by awarding bodies and approved by the NCVQ. At Foundation and Intermediate levels candidates take a total of nine units, at Advanced level they take 15. In addition there are core units concerned with number, communication and information technology. The GNVQs will be reviewed to keep them up to date with developments in the vocational area or in education but the following applies at Foundation, Intermediate and Advanced levels in September 1995 (NCVQ, 1995).

At Foundation level the three mandatory units are:

1. Understanding health and well-being (Foundation);
2. Understanding personal development (Foundation);
3. Investigating working in health and social care (Foundation).

There are four mandatory units in the GNVQ in Health and Social Care at Intermediate level and they are:

1. Promoting health and well-being (Intermediate);
2. Influences on health and well-being (Intermediate);
3. Health and social care services (Intermediate);
4. Communication and inter-personal relationships in health and social care (Intermediate).

At the Advanced level there are eight mandatory units:

1. Equal opportunities and individuals' rights (Advanced);
2. Inter-personal interaction in health and social care (Advanced);
3. Physical aspects of health and social well-being (Advanced);
4. Psycho-social aspects of health and social well-being (Advanced)
5. Structure and development of health and social care services (Advanced);
6. Health and social care practice (Advanced);
7. Educating for health and social well-being (Advanced);
8. Research perspectives in health and social care (Advanced).

National Vocational Qualifications (NVQs) in Care, which are competence-based vocational qualifications, also maintain a cross-discipline, cross-agency health and social care perspective at least up to level 3. Students and candidates for professional training programmes who emerge from the NVQ/GNVQ routes are likely to start from a whole sector perspective. This may be different in kind from the GCSE, A-level route and may lead to different choices in higher education modules and pathways if such choices are indeed available.

CREDITS AND MODULES

Some further/higher education institutions are experimenting with forms of course organisation which lead to multiple academic and professional outcomes, for example the University of the South Bank and the University of Portsmouth offer academic degrees with both social work and nursing outcomes. Others are also experimenting with cross-disciplinary and professional studies sometimes in modules.

The Higher Education Quality Council report referred to earlier 'Choosing to Change' makes some interesting points about the shift from courses to modules and credits which bear on this trend.

The report acknowledges that the case for courses is that they provide indispensable ingredients for students which cannot easily be replaced, ingredients such as:

- *Intellectual integrity*   a sense of intellectual unity . . . as students engage with the protocols of a subject discipline;
- *Intellectual rigour*   . . . students are . . . assessed in the totality of what they have learned rather than in sub-units . . .
- *Intellectual identity*   . . . students locate themselves . . . as medical, physics or history students
- *Public trust*   . . . the extent to which people generally and employers specifically 'know what they are getting' with a course.

Credit systems however are held to be better than courses at delivering access, achievement, flexibility, self-reliance and, interestingly from the point of view of this chapter, inter-disciplinarity.

A categorisation of disciplinary flexibility is also offered in 'Choosing to Change'. The categorisation is designed to 'distinguish between the propensity of disciplines to be made available to incoming students', and distinguishes disciplines as:

1. *Linear technical*   'such as natural sciences and engineering, which require technical competence upon which to build subsequent progression but which can tolerate limited engagement with sub-elements of disciplines';
2. *Linear consultative*   such as languages and mathematics, which involve progressive improvement throughout the course and which may have difficulty making later stages available to non-disciplinary students;
3. *Linear practical*   such as art and design, which cannot easily be subdivided for the purposes of intermediate entry within a credit system (that is, a student cannot do 'a bit of sculpture').
4. *Discourse dependent*   such as philosophy, some social sciences and some humanities, which require the development of a shared discourse to vitalise the discipline but which may make sub-elements available to outsiders;
5. *Discourse tolerant*   'such as some social sciences, some humanities, some business and law which can tolerate some lack of comprehensive engagement with internal discourses'.
(p. 324)

111

These descriptions are of academic disciplines not professions, but most of the professions active in health and social care would, through their professional associations and regulatory bodies, probably describe themselves as linear-technical or discourse-dependent and would wish to guard the rigour and integrity of their basic professional training and induction programmes specifying the length of training and the components. The experience of those trying to organise joint or shared learning during programmes of professional training shows how difficult it can be to work around or through regulatory bodies concerned with single disciplines or professions because the tendency, perhaps understandably, is to concentrate on that discipline or profession alone. The tendency, however, may result in the failure to grasp or make opportunities to further interprofessional understanding in basic professional programmes. Davidson and Lucas (1995) suggest that the UK could learn from experience in Scandinavia and Australia where greater progress has been made in multiprofessional education.

POSTGRADUATE

At postgraduate and post-qualifying level the picture in the UK is more optimistic. Storrie (1992), for example, contacted 15 Masters-level courses 'for professionally qualified health and social care practitioners which focus, at least in part, on increasing interprofessional understanding and co-operation and which establish a course content to enable people from different professional backgrounds to learn together'. Storrie grouped the courses into four categories according to whether the primary focus was:

1. A particular client group;
2. Care delivery;
3. Planning, organisation and management of services;
4. Interprofessional working.

Twenty-one different programmes were analysed and of these 11 focused on a particular client group, four on care delivery, three on planning, organisation and management of services, two on interprofessional working, and one (Medical Social Anthropology) was in the category 'other'. Storrie makes the point that most of the programmes were concerned to increase professional knowledge and understanding of client groups or care delivery and that interest in interprofessional working follows rather than leads these objectives. With the increased interest in continuing professional development, perhaps greater opportunities will be available to those organising and participating in the various types of interprofessional or multiprofessional training.

TYPES OF TRAINING, LEARNING AND EDUCATION

Storrie shows that some courses are designed to help people from various professions to advance knowledge and understanding of a mutually interesting useful topic such as a client group or a service. Others might set out deliberately to:

- help people develop the skills of working across professions to provide a coordinated multiprofessional service of some kind; or
- develop new perspectives, knowledge and skills through merging or sharing insights and experiences across professions and disciplines.

Clarke (1993), for example, argues that interdisciplinary programmes of learning, development or practice should lead to significant cognitive and ethical change, and that the success of interdisciplinary or interprofessional (as opposed to multiprofessional or multidisciplinary) activity should be measured by the extent to which it does lead to such change. Clarke argues '. . . the mastering of the basic "cognitive maps" of other professions is one of the hallmarks of inter-disciplinary experience . . . The cognitive map represents the entire conceptual framework used by a discipline, including its basic concepts, problem definitions, modes of enquiry, types of dissertation and explanation and general ideas about what represents a discipline' (Petrie, 1976). Similarly 'Interdisciplinary experiences must further growth in the recognition by their participants that value orientations vary across the professions and that their differences reveal significant information about the origin and nature of their responsibilities toward others including other professionals as well as the patient or client.'

Opportunities for interdisciplinary education and experience could be made available within all the stages and at all the levels in careers in health and social care. Clearly for most practitioners participation in such experiences will lead to more informed individual practice and better teamwork, although for some it will lead to new working practice, new insights and new forms of service. The arguments are extended in the next chapter to include service-user perspectives and recent developments in community care.

References

Clarke, P. G. (1993) A typology of interdisciplinary education in gerontology and geriatrics: 'are we really doing what we say we are'. *Journal of Interprofessional Care*, 7(3) pp. 217–27.

Clifton, M., with Thompson, T. and Brown, J. (1994) *Training and Education in Transition: Bridging Vocational and Academic Models in an Interdisciplinary Perspective*' York: University of York MHNA.

Davidson, L. and Lucas, J. (1995) Multi-professional education in the undergraduate health professions curriculum: observations from Adelaide, Linkoping and Salford. *Journal of Interprofessional Care*, 9(2), August 1995.

Dearing, R. (1996) Review of Qualifications for 16–19 year olds. Summary Report, SCAA – School Curriculum and Assessment Authority, SCAA Middlesex.

Higher Education Quality Council (HEQC) (1994) *Choosing to Change. Extending access, choice and mobility in higher education*. The report of the HEQC (CAT Project). London: HEQC.

Joint Awarding Bodies (JAB) 1993 *Professional and Occupational Standards in the Care Sector*. Report of the Awarding Bodies and the Care Sector Consortium Conference. Available from JAB, Derbyshire House, St Chad's Street, London WC1.

National Council for Vocational Qualifications (NCVQ) (1995) *General National Vocational Qualifications, Mandatory Units for Advanced Health and Social Care* and *Mandatory Units for Intermediate Health and Social Care*. London: NCVQ.

National Council for Vocational Qualifications (NCVQ) *Monitor*, Summer 1995, p. 22.

Petrie, H. G. (1976) Do you see what I see? The epistemology of interdisciplinary inquiry. *Journal of Aesthetic Education*, 10, pp. 29–43.

Schon, D. A. (1992) The crisis of professional knowledge and the pursuit of an epistemology of practice. *Journal of Interprofess-*

ional Care, 6(1) Spring, pp. 48–65. Reproduced from Christensson, C. R. with Hansen, A. J. (eds) (1987), *Teaching by the Case Method*, Boston, Mass: Harvard Business School.

Storrie, J. (1992) Mastering interprofessionalism – an enquiry into the development of Masters Programmes with an interprofessional focus. *Journal of Interprofessional Care* 6(3) Autumn pp. 253–9.

Preparation for Interprofessional Work: Holism, Integration and the Purpose of Training and Education

Peter Mathias, Ruth Prime and Tony Thompson

INTRODUCTION

The purpose of this chapter is to:

1. Identify the implications of the part played by people who use the services in achieving unified and integrated programmes of health and social care – one of the key goals of interprofessional working;
2. Examine the implications of recent developments in community care for learning and training;
3. Explore briefly the ideas of holism in health and social practice and the ideas of differentation and integration in the professions to help think about the purpose and nature of interprofessional programmes of learning.

HOLISM

Lämsä, Hietanen and Lämsä (1994) describe how the reform of the Finnish educational system allows for a systematic approach to education for holistic care and holistic professionalism. Their argument is that the separation of professions in health care and social work has led to unhelpful fragmentation in services and in education. Holism is seen to extend to economic understanding and wider participation of professions in society. The pilot programme they describe, which is designed to help young people move into careers in the health and social services is firmly based on a platform of joint vocational studies.

Similarly on the theme of holism, Frederick (1995) argues that holistic approaches embrace, integrate and unify diverse efforts of care givers, and that professionals should be alert to the sort of 'destructive separation' from other professionals which can damage the holistic treatment of patients or the holistic provision of care.

Damaging and destructive separation of professionals, one from the other and from the patient's or client's world, including their world of help and support, is often associated with poor practice and poor health or social outcomes and also often associated with an equally damaging and destructive separation of one agency from another.

Separation may involve the cognitive maps, and values of Clarke, mentioned in the previous chapter. It may involve patterns of communication and creativity of decision-making and it may be influenced and mediated by the power, responsibility and status of the various participants.

Integration of professional activity will seek to bring together various types of intervention and support into a balanced programme of health or social care sensitive to the physical, the psychological, the educational, the social and the spiritual. To be successful, interprofessional activity or practice should not be separated from the client or service user.

PATIENTS, CLIENTS OR SERVICE USERS: ACTIVE CONTRIBUTORS

If one of the purposes of interprofessional working is the combining of different perspectives into a programme which results in health or social gain, then the patients or service users are interprofessional workers *par excellence* as in the vast majority of cases it is they (perhaps with the support of the primary care grouping) who unify and combine different advice and perspectives integrating them into daily living and making health choices as they do so. How do they do it, and can training and learning help?

117

Previously (Mathias, 1991) it was argued that descriptions and definitions of the various professional and non-professional help and support systems are useful when thinking about interprofessional working, because they serve to place it in context and because they offer a slightly different set of answers to those which usually apply to questions about how to increase interprofessional effectiveness in health and social care. Some of these arguments will be repeated and extended here.

Sugarman (1986) argues that people turn to a hierarchy of support, ranging from the formal to the informal, when faced with major problems of one sort or another and these can be taken to include problems of health and social care. More specifically, Sugarman identifies the range of support to include (1) the natural help system, (2) the mutual help system, (3) the non-professional help system and (4) the professional help system.

Natural help system

The natural help or kith and kin system is often the first line of help and consists of people in the immediate network, although of course, sometimes, for a variety of reasons, the immediate network may be unhelpful and to be avoided. The decision to seek help and then where to seek it from is heavily influenced by individual experience and the advice of friends and family, as indeed is the response to help offered and advice provided.

The decisions and discussions about the type of problem experienced and how and from whom help can best be obtained is often heavily influenced by local knowledge, this general practitioner (GP) usually adopts such and such an approach: '. . . those social services offices usually take the line . . . this hospital consultant doesn't believe in . . .' So from the beginning those using the services (with some exceptions) are active in selecting the source of help, filtering the advice and organising a programme of health and social care which will vary in the range of professions involved according to the nature of the problem, the personality and beliefs of the user, and the views and characteristics of their immediate help system.

Byrne, Cunningham and Sloper (1988), for example, carried out a longitudinal study with a cohort of 181 families of children with Down's syndrome. They found that 23 per cent of families were in contact with five or more professionals, 56 per cent between 2 and 5, 14 per cent with one, and only 6 per cent were not in contact with any.

Disability, long-term illness or social deprivation often brings people into contact with a variety of professionals who have to be dealt with over longish periods of time. More acute problems may bring more rapid contact but commonly the user has to sift and weigh advice, make choices between the different suggestions and opinions and have the discipline to follow programmes of activity.

The argument here is that this often makes the user an inter-professional worker in the sense that they are better served if (i) they have the skills and confidence to draw the best out of different professionals, (ii) they have a basic grounding and understanding of the health or social problem they experience and its various 'professional' dimensions, and (iii) they have the confidence and skills to make choices and decisions.

The extent to which people are able to do these things effectively will vary according to circumstance. Byrne, Cunningham and Sloper report two themes in their study. The first is family variety, normality and strength; the second is vulnerability. Vulnerable families included those with serious health problems, with children with more severe learning difficulties, and those coping with unemployment and/or poor parental education. If interprofessional work is to be effective it would well recognise:

1. that in the majority of cases it is the service user who combines different sources of advice into a unified programme, and
2. that users are made better or less able to do this by factors which heighten or lessen vulnerability such as severity and range of problem(s), their educational background, strength of voice and the attitudes, competence and state of knowledge of the professions involved.

Education and training can make interprofessional work more effective in these instances by influencing both user and profes-sional. Programmes, whether general or specific, designed to give knowledge to and increase the skills of the service user will result in more effective care, particularly if they help the user make use of and integrate ideas from different professions. Similarly, profes-sionals might be helped to work together to look at the local opportunities for various types of patient or client.

The mutual help system and the non-professional help system

Sugarman's analysis of the hierarchy of support leads to a consideration of how the mutual help and the non-professional help systems might also contribute to the effectiveness of interprofessional working.
Bean (1975) identifies three types of mutual help groups:

1. Those organised around a particular crisis, for example the death of a child;
2. Those for people with a permanent condition subject to stigma and disadvantage; and
3. Those for people caught in a habit, addiction or self-destructive way of life.

Mutual help groups may offer support and/or act as pressure groups for the improvement of services and may well enable people to develop the skill and expertise to make effective use of different sources of advice.

From such groups may also spring those who guide others through the maze of services and often confusing variety of approaches to health and social care issues and problems. The usefulness of such activity was recognised in the Report of the Committee of Enquiry into the Education of Handicapped Children and Young People. Special Educational Needs (1978). The report contained a proposal for a named person to help parents, particularly those of young children with special needs, to find their way through the variety of services and professionals.

The responsibility for guiding and helping to interpret advice from different helping professions often falls on those in the non-professional help system. Golan (1981) argues that the non-professional help system consists of voluntary workers, community care givers and para-professionals. Teachers, police officers and clergy are included in the middle category because they are people who are in direct contact with various client groups, but whose qualifications are not specifically in helping.

Professional help and recent developments in community care

A number of professionals find themselves in jobs in which they are called on to coordinate and obtain advice from different sources and translate it into a programme of activity with, or on behalf of, a client. Many management posts carry this responsibility and it is also a feature of basic activity for some social workers, teachers, nurses and doctors.

'Examples of this are the head teacher who convenes a multi-disciplinary group of speech and physiotherapists and social workers in order to respond to the needs of pupils; the ward manager who has to translate the advice of doctors, psychologists and paramedical specialists (professions allied to medicine) into daily programmes of activities for patients and the day services worker who arranges or helps to arrange a programme including different disciplines in order to help a client overcome particular difficulties.'

(Mathias, 1991)

Case management and care management are particular and more formal examples of the way of thinking.

Interprofessional working is often associated with teams, but if we allow ourselves to take a lateral look at the idea it becomes apparent that a variety of people, including the user, patient or client, are active in using or combining advice and help and therefore contribute to interprofessional effectiveness measured in terms of integration of programmes of health and social care in individual instances.

THE INTEGRATION OF HEALTH AND SOCIAL CARE

In its policy evidence to the 1989 White Paper, *Caring for People: Community Care in the Next Decade and Beyond*, the Department of Health defines community care as 'the provision of services which people who are affected by problems of ageing, mental illness, mental handicap or physical or sensory disability need to be able to live as independently a life as possible in their own homes or in homely settings in the community'.

The same document defines 'collaboration' as a 'partnership of joint working between all authorities and agencies involved in planning and delivering community services'.

The aims and objectives of interprofessional working and practice can therefore be defined as the coming together of people from different professions and disciplines, each having specialist knowledge and skills,

- to give and share information,
- determine needs,
- formulate plans and
- provide appropriate care,

to enable the individual(s) to live the highest quality of life and enjoy the maximum independence possible in the community. In essence, interprofessional practice is an integral aspect of holistic care.

The White Paper, Caring for People (1989), in its discussion of Principles of Assessment states: 'Some individuals will suffer not from a single problem or disability but from several, covering both social and health care needs. In these cases no single professional discipline can encompass the whole picture. The assessment procedure will therefore need to be flexible enough to take as broad a view as possible.'

The text continues:

'all agencies and professionals involved with the individual and his or her problem should be brought into the assessment procedure when necessary. These include social workers, GPs, community nurses, hospital staff such as consultants in geriatric medicine, psychiatry, rehabilitation and other hospital specialists, nurses, physiotherapists, occupational therapists, speech therapists, continence advisers, community psychiatric nurses, staff involved in vision and hearing, housing officers, the Employment Department's Resettlement and Employment Rehabilitation Service, home helps, home care assistants and voluntary workers.'

This is indeed a very impressive and somewhat daunting list of possible participants, but the important point, as stated, is that people should be involved when necessary, in other words when they have a pertinent contribution to make.

Inherent problems

Professionals working together, while highly desirable and vitally important, does not in itself guarantee that the desired outcome will be achieved. Inherent in this style of working are understandable problems which need to be acknowledged and guarded against if communication is to be effective and a positive outcome achieved.

Training activities will have to address the problems in one way or another. The problematic areas include:

- understanding the purpose of interprofessional practice;
- understanding the role of others;
- professional rivalry;
- exclusion of the significant others (non-professionals);
- ownership of resources;
- discrimination and racism; and
- making sure that assessment is effective.

Understanding the purpose of interprofessional practice

It is of the utmost importance that every participant clearly understands that this method of working as already stated is first and foremost for the benefit of the individual(s) in need. It is not a forum for people to display knowledge or vie for status or engage in professional rivalry.

Kenneth Calman (1994) in his article 'Working together: teamwork', states 'The shared aims of a team are obviously important but do not occur by spontaneous generation. They need to be hammered out, discussed and debated and by joint agreement put into practice'.

Understanding the role of others

Interprofessional practice necessitates interaction between professionals at various levels – group discussion, telephone communication and written communication among others. Each individual has a different role to play but it cannot be assumed that each person understands the role of others. Clarification of roles from the onset is necessary. Failure to do so can lead to confusion, tension and rivalry.

Professional rivalry

In some settings there may be an hierarchical structure and deference and respect is based on the position in the hierarchy. In others a very different structure may operate, and workers of varying responsibilities may interact on a more equal basis. When a number of people from different disciplines come together, each used to working in different structures and having different expectations, it is not surprising if members in various ways come to feel that their contribution is not given the status they think it deserves.

Interprofessional practice is not, however, to do with hierarchy of role or hierarchy of importance; it is a partnership in which everyone's contribution is of equal importance and each person has a distinctive role to play.

The Barclay Report (1982) states 'collaboration between workers social workers and other services should be on a basis of mutual respect . . . arrangements for collaboration need to be planned and factors which affect relationships need to be understood and not give rise to tension by both managers and practitioners'.

Exclusion of significant others

There is a danger that professionals may seem so preoccupied with professionalism or role that they are likely to forget that patients or clients, their carers and other relevant people in their lives have a significant contribution to make. Needs cannot be properly defined or appropriately met without the involvement of all those others. This sentiment is expressed in the White Paper, *Caring for People* – assessment should take account of the wishes of the individual and their carer and of the carer's ability to continue to provide care and where possible include their active participation. Good community care will take account of the circumstances of minority communities and will be planned in consultation with others.

Discrimination and racism

Discrimination against people on the grounds of age, sex, religion, sexual orientation, race and disability is prevalent throughout society. Professionals must therefore acknowledge that as part of a society which subscribes to discrimination they must examine their own bias and deal with it.

They must also be aware that racism is discrimination with added dimensions. Racism is the combined use of prejudice and power against people from black and minority ethnic communities. There is an abundance of evidence to prove that racism in the caring professions, as in other walks of life, deprives black and minority ethnic people of badly needed services. For example, Baxter (1992) provides an analysis of the effects of racism in providing care for people with a learning disability.

Michael Day (1994) argues that:

'Racism and discrimination are not confined to acts of hostility towards individuals or groups. The uncomfortable truth is that the most pervasive forms of discrimination and racism persist in systems and institutions. Cultures which are shaped by long tradition and where specialist skills are practised and entry restricted to the highly qualified can become professional enclaves. Like minded people reinforce shared perceptions and sustain working methods which are unresponsive to a changing environment.'

It is imperative, therefore, that all involved should undergo some form of training to assist them in understanding personal and institutional racism and how racist conditioning affects their feelings, perception and attitudes. Without this understanding it would be impossible to develop anti-racist strategies in the provision of services.

Earlier, the exclusion of significant others was discussed. Black representatives with relevant knowledge are significant others when dealing with black and minority ethnic people. The role of black representatives must be clear as should the strategies for the giving and sharing of information and ensuring that overt or covert racism does not operate.

Ownership of resources

Meeting needs determined by professionals can become a thorny issue largely because the professionals who own the resources may be faced with competing demands for those resources, rendering them unable to provide in full measure. The result may well be anger from the other professionals and resentment on their part. In periods of scarce resources that danger is even greater.

ASSESSMENT

Assessment is one of the greatest interprofessional concerns and challenges, the purpose of which is to determine whether there are factors where absence or presence may have caused problems or had adverse effects on the quality of life. Having identified these factors an evaluation is made, conclusions are drawn and decisions taken.

Professionals coming together share a great deal of information about the individual(s) and carer – physical health, environment, social situation, emotional state, financial situation, abilities, strengths and weaknesses, culture, impact of racism, lifestyle, interest, past history, recent crises and other issues. They also share information about the actual or probable impact the aforementioned may have on the individual, based on professional knowledge and skills. Individuals and carers also share their perceptions and wishes.

This wealth of information is meaningless unless evaluated as a whole. There is always a risk that decisions are made on isolated bits of information but this is a dangerous practice which must be avoided at all costs. Skills and objectivity are vital in the evaluation process and individuals and teams need practice in evaluating and analysing complex arrays of information.

After evaluation, decisions are made about how best to resolve problems and meet needs while allowing the individual to make maximum use of his or her abilities, and to enjoy the greatest level of independence possible. A care plan or package of care may now be drawn up stating quite clearly what is to be done, by whom and within what time limits.

Each participant can now contribute their skills and play an appropriate role. It does not follow that everyone involved in assessment will take an active role in intervention and support. The package must be designed to give the individual maximum help with minimum intrusion. Training must therefore equip practitioners to take part in assessment as well as in direct provision and in monitoring and review of the programme itself.

IMPLICATIONS

Interprofessional practice clearly has implications for workers, managers, trainers, clients and carers.

By and large, workers are most comfortable working with others of their own profession/discipline as they share the same goals, priorities and a familiar structure. Interprofessional practice and learning calls for an understanding of numerous aspects of other professions – mutual professional respect, honesty, and an ability to listen, willingness to learn and a preparedness to deal with racist and discriminatory attitudes. Workers, therefore, need to work at interprofessional practice and to be assisted by managers who must have the commitment and will to provide the framework within which professionals can operate effectively.

Preparation for interprofessional practice should begin at an early stage. Students should be educated about this style of working and training should involve the issues raised in this chapter. Indeed there is a case for some aspects of training to be undertaken jointly by different professionals. Training does not, however, end once a qualification has been acquired, it should continue in the workplace and when necessary through attending courses. A good example is training for managing the process.

Participation by clients and carers must be both encouraged and facilitated. Managers must make certain that they are kept informed about the department's policies and practice and understand what is going on.

Health and social needs are so inextricably related that no one profession can adequately meet the needs of all individuals. Educational and training programmes, from general health promotion and advocacy to highly specific and targeted programmes on particular health or social topics, play a part in increasing interprofessional effectiveness.

Planning learning

Clarke (1993) reminds us that in devising opportunities for learning we should be clear about the objectives, pay attention to method and be realistic about time.

There may be many different types of programmes in the field of interprofessional learning including:

1. those programmes or activities which are designed to help professionals and practitioners of one profession to work constructively with those of another, in order to integrate or unify health and social care programmes so that they are sensitive to client or user situations;
2. those programmes which are designed to create new thinking, to set new problems, and to design new services;
3. efforts to increase the involvement and develop the expertise of users and people active in the non-professional help system.

Frederick (1995) observes that 'Western civilisation has been preoccupied with understanding unity and multiplicity or 'the one and the many from time immemorial' arguing that there is both a tendency towards greater and greater differentiation as organisations evolve, and another tendency towards cooperation, centripetal organisation and integration.

The proliferation of specialist, highly differentiated professions and the equal call for interprofessionalism, for sharing and for integration reflects this preoccupation. The tension between the highly differentiated and the integrated is also reflected in Checkland's (1981) book on systems thinking. He presses the case for interdisciplinary theories which can 'point out similarities between the theoretical constructions of different disciplines, reveal gaps in empirical knowledge and provide a language by means of which experts in different disciplines could communicate with each other' (p. 108).

In a similar vein, Schon (1987) comments that professionals in America in the 1970s were beginning to become aware of 'the indeterminate zones of practice the situations of complexity and uncertainty, the unique cases that require artistry, the elusive lack of problem setting, the multiplicity of professional identity'.

Schon reminds us to be aware of the multiplicity within a single profession, and that there are likely to be competing and complementary schools of thought within single disciplines. It can also be true that practitioners of branches of one profession may have more in common with practitioners of the same branch of other professions than with colleagues in the same profession. Professions also change, re-organise, split, merge and otherwise respond to changes in their environment.

As well as the issues discussed in this chapter a number of other factors will constrain or determine the nature of individual interprofessional exercises, some of which are explored in other chapters of this book. For example, Simon Biggs in Chapter 9 offers further clarification of terms and examines the implications of recent British legislation and social policy. Jenny Weinstein in Chapter 7 analyses and draws lessons from the Joint Practice Teaching Initiative. Margaret Coats and Lindsay Mitchell describe the development of the Functional Map of Health and Social Care in Chapter 8, and Tony Thompson and Peter Mathias in Chapter 10 examine the implications of the policies of the World Health Organisation and European Union for cooperation amongst professionals.

References

Barclay Report (1982) *Social Workers: Their Roles and Tasks.* London: Bedford Square Press.

Baxter, C. (1992) Providing care in a multi-racial society. in T. Thompson, and P. Mathias, (eds), *Standards and Mental Handicap: Keys to Competence.* London: Baillière Tindall.

Bean, M. (1975) Alcoholics anonymous part II. *Psychiatric Annals*, pp. 317–57.

Boulding, K. E. (1956) 'General systems theory – the skeleton of science. *Management Science*, 2 (3).

Byrne, E. A., Cunningham, C., Sloper, P., (1988) *Families and their Children with Down's Syndrome: One Feature in Common.* London: Routledge.

Calman, K. (1994) Working together: teamwork'. *Journal of Interprofessional Care*, vol 8(1) pp. 95–9.

'Caring for People: Community Care in Next Decade and Beyond,' London: HMSO, CM 849: 1989.

Checkland, P. (1981) *Systems Thinking, Systems Practice.* Chichester: John Wiley.

Clarke, P. G. (1993) A typology of interdisciplinary education in gerontology and geriatrics: 'are we really doing what we say we are'. *Journal of Inter-Professional Care*, 7(3) pp. 217–27.

Clifton, M., Thompson, T. and Brown, J. (1994) *Training and Education in Transition: Bridging Vocational and Academic Models in an Interdisciplinary Perspective.* York: University of York MHNA.

Day, M. (1994) Racial Discrimination; Professional Implications. *Journal of Interprofessional Care*, 8(2) pp. 135–40.

Department of Health (1989) *Caring for People: Community Care in the Next Decade and Beyond.* Cm 849. London: HMSO.

Frederick, C. (1995) A holographic approach to holism. *Journal of Interprofessional Care* 9(1) pp. 9–15.

Golan, N. (1981) *Passing through Transitions: A Guide for Practitioners.* New York: Free Press.

Lamsa, A., Hietanen, I. and Lamsa, J. (1994) Education for holistic care: a pilot programme in Finland. *Journal of Interprofessional Care* (international issue), 8(1) Spring.

Mathias, P. (1991) Multidisciplinary care and training. In R. C. McGillivray and A. M. Green (eds), *Hallas' Caring for People with Mental Handicaps*, 8th edn. London: Butterworth-Heinemann.

129

Petrie, H. G. (1976) Do you see what I see? The epistemology of interdisciplinary inquiry. *Journal of Aesthetic Education*, 10, (pp. 29–43).

Report of the Committee of Enquiry into the Education of Handicapped Children and Young People. Special Educational Needs (Warnock Report) HMSO Cmnd 7212: 1978.

Schon, D. A. (1992) The crisis of professional knowledge and the pursuit of an epistemology of practice. In *Journal of Interprofessional Care*, 6(1) Spring, pp. 48–65.

Sugarman, L. (1986) *Life Span Development: Concepts, Theories and Interventions* London: Methuen.

CHAPTER SEVEN

The Development of Shared Learning: Conspiracy or Constructive Development?

Jenny Weinstein

INTRODUCTION

The purpose of this chapter is twofold. The focus is an innovative project developed between 1990 and 1995 to encourage the joint training of practice teachers/clinical supervisors in nursing, occupational therapy and social work. On one level, it is hoped that this analysis of the project will provide a useful model for those interested in organising joint training programmes. On another level the project serves as a case study to illustrate some of the changes in the roles and status of health care professionals, the moving boundaries between them, and the interface between these changes and current developments in professional education and training.

The progress of the Joint Practice Teaching Initiative is charted identifying issues and learning points at three key stages. From the outset, in spite of considerable enthusiasm and an apparently positive context, the problems which were to beset the project began to emerge. At the midway point, the failure to achieve jointly validated programmes was investigated and the barriers identified. By the end, strategies for overcoming the barriers had been developed and further contextual changes gave an additional boost to the success and extension of the project.

The barriers themselves and the strategies for overcoming them were associated with a range of political, social and educational themes. These related in various ways to demands for radical reform of the professions and the welfare state from both Left and Right (Johnson, 1972; Illich, 1977; Hayek, 1960; Minford, 1987). While increased competition and the struggle for survival in the welfare market appeared to unite professionals in some respects, in others they exacerbated 'tribalism' and defensiveness. The significant enhancement of employers' influence through increased financial control of professional education and the new emphasis on service user involvement were found to pose both threats and opportunities for the promotion of shared learning. Undoubtedly the most controversial development was the government's policy to establish common occupational standards from which Scottish/National Vocational Qualifications (S/NVQs) at levels 4 and 5 (equivalent to professional level) could be derived. Enthusiasts for demystifying professional expertise and redrawing professional boundaries welcomed these developments (Ellis, 1988; Hevey, 1992); others, who saw it as a strategy to dilute the professions, were very suspicious about the motives for encouraging joint training (Webb, 1992).

THE PROJECT

The Joint Practice Teaching Initiative (referred to here as JPTI or the joint initiative) was established in 1989 when the Central Council for Education and Training in Social Work (CCETSW) provided £30 000 a year, over five years, to develop joint training for practice teachers/clinical supervisors in health and welfare. The project is significant because of the key role which practice teachers and clinical supervisors play as the trainers and socialisers of the next generation of professionals within the work context. Students from all caring professions are likely to rate their practice/clinical experience as the most valued aspect of their training. The practice/clinical placement links the student and the education institution with new developments in practice while practice teachers/clinical supervisors are linked back to the educational institution and to current issues about education and training.

JPTI is studied in relation to the various systems with which it is inextricably linked. Hunter and Wistow (1987, pp. 15–16) identify three levels at which such systems operate:

132

- National or interdepartmental level;
- Local or inter-agency level;
- Field or interprofessional level.

At the national level, the project involved negotiations between professional bodies about validation and statutory requirements. It was also operating within the context of the government's imperative to develop occupational standards in the health and care sectors, and was influenced by the controversy about taking National Vocational Qualifications to level 5, professional level (Department of Employment, 1995).

At the local level the project was affected by changes in service delivery, changes in higher education, changes in the content and delivery of pre-and post-registration training for all three professions, and changes in the way education was being funded following Working Paper 10 (DH, 1989a).

At the field or interprofessional level the project encountered practical problems about timetables and venues, as well as more profound problems about culture, values and professional norms which had to be defined and negotiated between project participants.

The aims and objectives for JPTI were not specified by the Department of Health and the project was not linked to any particular policy initiative, apart from the unspecified promotion of joint training in documents such as the White Paper, *Caring for People* (DH, 1989b, p. 67):

'It will be important to continue to develop multi-disciplinary training for staff in all caring professions . . .'

and the Government guidance on child protection, *Working Together* (DH, 1991):

'It is recommended that agencies should establish joint annual training programmes . . .'

The project was initiated and managed by CCETSW to further its stated objective to encourage multidisciplinary training and to contribute to the training of other professions. Over the five years, JPTI was piloted on 12 sites across the UK, and five jointly-validated programmes were run and evaluated in England.

EVALUATION OF THE PROJECT

It is always difficult to devise a means of evaluating a developmental project. By their very nature such projects evolve as they are influenced by their rapidly-changing context. For this reason, JPTI was evaluated using an action research approach. This model is specifically concerned with the management of change. It recognises a feedback loop between the objectives of the project, the intervention of the researchers, the action of the participants, the impact of the immediate environment and the further direction of the project. Torbert (in Reason and Rowan, 1981, p. 143) points out that where most practitioners are operating in a context of constant turmoil, it is difficult to establish rigorous experimental research conditions in which variables are kept constant and controlled.

The project was evaluated at different stages and in a range of ways. All the pilot joint courses were asked to evaluate their experiences, to write them up and to report on them. Their findings were shared with colleagues at four workshops held during the five years of the project's life. The quality and length of project reports varied considerably and attempts to obtain write-ups in a common format were unsuccessful. Nevertheless, useful themes and issues emerged.

After the first year an independent researcher undertook an evaluation of the first four pilots. This was published by CCETSW (Brown, S., 1993). After the second year, the project manager undertook an in-depth retrospective investigation with the specific aim of identifying the barriers which were impeding the successful implementation of joint programmes (Weinstein, 1993). Finally, during the last 18 months, two project workers were appointed to support the pilots, to undertake a further evaluation. A final report was published by CCETSW (Bartholomew *et al.*, 1996).

None of the researchers can claim complete objectivity. Even the independent researcher found himself drawn into the role of consultant and supporter of the pilots, although this had not been the intention of his brief. With respect to reliability and external validity, the criteria claimed for this research are those identified by Lincoln (1985) as credibility, transferability, dependability and confirmability. The collaborative paradigm, described by Reason and Rowan (1981, p. 142) facilitates the exchange of ideas, knowledge, views and understanding required to progress this kind of initiative. The JPTI evaluation relied on the findings of the different

134

researchers from their different perspectives being similar and making sense to steering-group members and other interested parties. These findings also coincided with those of researchers studying similar joint training projects (Walton, 1989; Brown, 1994).

STAGE 1 – ESTABLISHMENT OF PILOTS AND THE DEVELOPMENT OF THE CORE MODULE

In January 1990, CCETSW consulted representatives from relevant education bodies about the viability of joint training for practice teachers from different professions.. A positive response provided the impetus to establish an interprofessional steering group which consisted of representatives from the English National Board for Nursing, Midwifery and Health Visiting (ENB), the College of Occupational Therapists (COT) and an interprofessional group of educationalists. The core members of this group have steered JPTI for four and a half years on an informal basis without remuneration.

JPTI was launched with a large workshop in September 1990 attended by over 80 delegates from social work, nursing and occupational therapy. The purpose was to test the water prior to initiating pilot projects. The conference was a success in terms of being oversubscribed and stimulating a high level of participation by those who attended. The issues raised were clearly controversial, arousing considerable 'storming' before reaching a consensus on the way forward. The proceedings were permeated by a number of key themes which came to dominate the project throughout its life:

- There were very few managers or purchasers at the conference. Failure to get them on board at the beginning proved an ongoing problem throughout the project.
- Everyone was very enthusiastic about the idea of shared learning. People enjoyed the small groups discussions and were delighted to find out how much they had in common. There was no doubt about the commonalities in the roles of practice teachers/clinical supervisors from the different professions.
- But there was also a lot of suspicion. Whose idea was this? Did it come from the government? If it did, what was the hidden agenda? Were we selling out on the preservation of unique

professions? Were we selling out on the quality of service to users?

- Time featured as a major concern. Although there was support for the idea in principle, where would people find the time to organise such a venture in the current climate of change? Perhaps they would think about it when things settled down a little.
- Participants were concerned about the role of the validating bodies. Had they got their act together yet to sort out how joint validation would work? Seeking validation from one body was already back-breaking, without having to meet requirements of a further two or three.

Nevertheless, the outcome on the whole was positive and some practical proposals for future action emerged:

- To produce a glossary of terms in order to improve communication and reduce misunderstandings between the professions;
- To undertake more detailed work to identify the common competences for practice teachers and those which are unique to each profession;
- For the professional education bodies to clarify processes for validation of joint courses;
- To build on existing local and national collaborative links;
- To produce and distribute a workshop report to all participants and other interested parties.

                                                              (CCETSW, 1990)

All conference participants were given application forms to tender for pump-priming money to initiate pilot projects for joint-practice teacher-training. The criteria for tenders were that the pilots would be genuinely collaborative ventures between health and social services; that they would be underpinned by the anti-racist and anti-discriminatory value-base of JPTI; and that they would provide a full progress report of their activities to the steering group after one year.

Four projects were funded in the first instance and their leaders came together at a workshop held in Birmingham in September 1991. Representatives from each project made interesting presentations about their progress to date which were recorded in the workshop report (CCETSW, 1991). These indicated considerable enthusiasm in the field for joint training in spite of a large number of practical problems and some concern about the possible impact on 'professional identity'. Participants listed what they saw as positive and negative features of joint training from their experience so far. The lists were fairly evenly balanced. On the positive side, they included:

- Better services for the consumer;
- United by adversity and strength through sharing;
- Better understanding of each other's roles by not training in a professional vacuum;
- Scope for creative thinking across boundaries;
- Maximised range and quality of resources;
- Enhanced teamwork;
- Cooperation as a power base for change.

On the negative side, they identified the following problems to overcome:

- Lack of basic infrastructure;
- Lack of shared meanings and definitions;
- Professional resistance, defence mechanisms and tribalism;
- Potential problems of quality control;
- The threat of uniformity;
- Fear of a hidden agenda which might lead to dilution of professions;
- Different approaches to race and disability.

Project leaders expressed considerable disappointment that, a year on from the conference, there had been no progress in developing joint validation procedures by the education bodies. Because of this, the steering group decided to use the grant for 1991/2 to fund a further tranche of pilots, using the same procedures and criteria as before. They also decided to commission an independent consultant to undertake a more systematic evaluation of the four pilot projects.

In the meantime, the working group which had been established in November 1990 to undertake the work on procedures for joint validation, was still struggling. The problems focused on an unwillingness to approve jointly validated programmes which would lead to all professionals receiving the same award. The English National Board for Nursing, Midwifery and Health Visiting was adamant that its awards, which involve registration, must be discrete. There were also problems about level, because community practice teachers in nursing oversee post-registration nurses while occupational therapy supervisors and social work practice teachers work with qualifying students.

The breakthrough came when agreement was reached to jointly validate a core module of practice teacher training which could be shared by all three professions (see Figure 7.1). However, this was on the understanding that each profession, having shared their learning on the module, would then go on to be assessed for, and receive a profession-specific award or qualification. As the components of the core module were already part of existing requirements for programmes from all three professions, the adoption of a shared learning approach could be viewed by the validating bodies as a 'modification' of existing approved programmes.

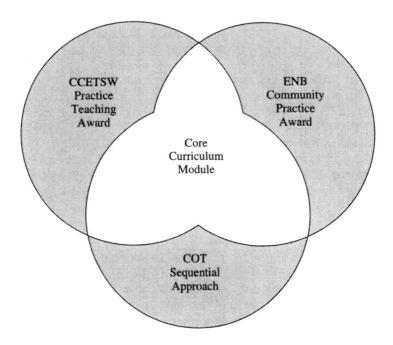

Figure 7.1   The JPTI core curriculum module developed in April 1992

Once this principle had been established, it was very easy for the relevant representatives from Occupational Therapy, Social Work and Nursing, Midwifery and Health Visiting, using the work of the pilot projects, to agree the content of a core module which derived from the common elements of the practice teaching programmes of the three professions. (CCETSW, 1989; COT, 1988; ENB, 1991). The key components of the core module were:

1. *Development of self as a practice teacher/clinical supervisor.* The candidate would

- undertake a self assessment of her/his potential as a practice teacher;
- learn to develop a practice curriculum relevant to own context knowledge and skills;
- explore the issues involved in teaching students to link theory and practice and to become reflective practitioners.

2. *Exploration of adult learning theories.* The candidate would

- consider a range of educational theories in relation to adult learning;
- gain an understanding of a variety of teaching and learning styles;
- learn how to help students identify their own learning needs and find appropriate ways to meet them.

3. *Achievement of skills in assessment.* The candidate would

- learn the difference between the assessment process and assessment events;
- learn to facilitate student participation in all aspects of the assessment process;
- identify good practice in dealing with failing and borderline students; and
- learn to write a comprehensive assessment report using specific evidence to demonstrate how the student has or has not met learning objectives.

In addition three 'value added' elements were introduced to enrich the core curriculum which were:

4. Equal opportunities and anti-racist and anti-discriminatory practice.
5. Professional collaboration in community care.
6. 'Long-arm' supervision (potential for placing a student from one profession in a placement supervised by another professional but with long-arm supervision from a practice teacher of his or her own profession).

The steering group decided that the workshop for the pilot projects for 1992 should consider the best ways of actually developing and running the core module. This workshop was clearly a step forward from the previous ones because it moved on from debating the pros and cons of joint training, and began to address good practice in actually establishing and running joint programmes.

The workshop was helped by a presentation from Steve Brown, the independent consultant, who reported on his initial findings with respect to the four first-year pilots. Brown (1993) identified the following indicators of effective joint training:

- The development of initiatives reflect the local concerns and priorities of service agencies, and training developments are linked with service strategies.
- Initiatives take place within a framework of collaboration between health and social services service agencies and education institutions.
- Key players from all the agencies and professions are involved and willing to agree about lead roles and tasks.
- Innovative joint approaches are encouraged and rewarded with clear incentives for agencies and professions to move forward together.

STAGE 2 – THE BARRIERS TO ACHIEVING JOINTLY VALIDATED PROGRAMMES

While the publication of the core curriculum, Brown's report and the very positive workshop gave considerable encouragement to the steering group, it soon became evident that the actual implementation of jointly-validated courses was much more problematic than had been anticipated.

While initially there were 18 responses to invitations to tender for funds to run the core module, one-third of the successful tenderers dropped out prior to signing the contract. Applicants were prepared to organise brief two or three day shared learning workshops, but withdrew when the project manager made it clear that funding was only available for a fully validated core module organised as part of an official practice teacher-training programme.

By November 1992, serious concern was being expressed about the future of the project. After three years of the project's existence, no fully collaborative programme for practice teachers had been validated, run and evaluated. The one programme which had been planned and was due to run in April 1993 had attracted only six students. The majority of trainee practice teachers in the region were pursuing their own profession-specific courses.

The project manager and the steering group undertook to try and identify the barriers to getting these programmes off the ground (Weinstein, 1993). The documentation on the first two years of the project was thoroughly examined. This comprised minutes of steering group meetings, three conference reports, tenders and reports from the pilots and correspondence. Meetings were held with representatives from projects, steering group members, and representatives from validating bodies. In addition, interviews were held with a 'control' group of 14 managers, practitioners and educationalists of the three professions, who were not involved with the project, to ascertain their views and experiences with respect to the value and practicality of organising joint training.

The outcome of the investigation was the identification of the following barriers to implementing the joint programmes:

- The absence of organisational and structural links with service planners or managers who are the purchasers of training and the employers of potential practice teachers;
- The impact of health, social services and education reforms which caused participants to prioritise the implementation of mainstream changes placed an innovative, experimental project on the back burner.
- An underlying fear that shared learning would lead to a further erosion of individual professions. This issue was linked closely to unresolved ethical and value conflicts between the professions.
- Insufficient time for planning programmes to meet interprofessional needs. The pump-priming money provided by CCETSW was not sufficient to employ someone to undertake the planning. Key participants were usually overwhelmed by other pressures.
- A lack of support for projects which were left isolated and marginalised. Those involved did not feel part of a wider network and this lessened the incentive to achieve the goals.
- The complex nature of the core module which might be described as a mini course within a course rather than a fully shared programme. This caused considerable organisational problems.

141

Far more flexible approaches were required from the validating bodies to make the module more accessible.

A number of other interesting and important findings emerged.

- While managers and practitioners were likely to spend more than 50 per cent of their time in interprofessional collaboration, educationalists spend less than 25 per cent of their time in such activities.
- Managers were more likely than practitioners or educationalists to focus on the role and the task rather than the particular professional demarcations and status.
- Practitioners feared that too much collaboration might lead to false expectations of the other professional, to 'dumping' work or to making referrals inappropriately. They were also concerned about boundaries. One health visitor reflected many responses when she said, 'my space and my job are being invaded'.
- Other problems identified were blaming; one profession dominating; conflicts of values on issues such as race, gender and confidentiality; or being confused about one's own professional identity.
- The majority of respondents expressed cynicism about the government's motives in encouraging joint training, seeing it as a mainly cost-cutting exercise. This was exemplified in a response from a manager who said, 'I don't think it's about quality I'm afraid. I think they want to squash us all down and make us the same because we're expensive as we are.'
- Joint training was perceived as being less problematic and less threatening when organised in the workplace at post qualifying level than in educational institutions at qualifying/pre-registration level.
- The majority of respondents and participants saw significant benefits to students on qualifying courses being placed in settings of another professional group.

STAGE 3 – OVERCOMING THE BARRIERS

Following discussion of these findings, the steering group had to decide whether or not it was worthwhile continuing with the JPTI project or whether it was 'ahead of its time' and should be put on ice for the time being. After a lengthy debate it was decided to continue

142

for a further year, since seven of the joint projects were still operating and had plans to provide programmes, albeit a year later than scheduled.

Instead of initiating new projects, the steering group decided to fund a development worker to nurture existing ones and encourage them to establish clear time scales and work plans which, it was hoped, might enable them to achieve jointly-validated programmes. The project worker would be asked to help projects to relate more closely with local service managers to secure their involvement and commitment to joint training programmes. A further part of the brief would be to facilitate networking between projects so that learning was maximised, to link with other joint training projects and organisations and to ensure promotion and publicity of the core module and the work of JPTI.

The contract to undertake the project work was advertised in the national press and brought a good response. The tender was won by two social workers on a job share basis, both of whom had considerable experience of interprofessional education, practice teaching, networking and consultancy activities. The development workers visited all the projects at least once, and in some cases three times. They saw their role as to ensure that the lessons learnt by one project were quickly shared with the others so that they could benefit from each other's experience.

Project planning groups used the workers for support and consultancy through long drawn out and sometimes frustrating planning and implementation processes. The development workers also linked with CCETSW Social Work Education Advisers and ENB officers, where appropriate.

In order to extend the successful networking between JPTI projects, the development workers initiated a Newsletter in May 1994 with a second edition published in November 1994. The projects responded enthusiastically to the Newsletter because it gave them an opportunity to publicise their achievements and widen their range of networks. The Newsletter unexpectedly developed a life of its own, being passed round between people interested in interprofessional education who had not previously heard of JPTI. The outcome was the compilation of an extensive mailing list and the strengthening of links between JPTI and other interprofessional projects.

The conclusions drawn by the development workers (Bartholomew *et al.*, 1996) reinforced the findings of Brown (1993) and Weinstein (1993) about barriers and ways of overcoming them. The key issues in relation to achieving viable joint programmes emphasised by the project workers were:

- First and foremost, the importance of the joint approach becoming the mainstream approach for training practice teachers. Where initiatives had been undertaken on a one-off basis, even if they were successful, they did not outlive the pump-priming grant.
- Secondly the amount of time which is necessary for the initial planning and organisation of joint initiatives.
- Thirdly, successful projects were usually led by enthusiastic and determined leaders committed to change and willing to give considerable commitment.

Although, even by March 1995, not all the joint programmes had run a full course or been fully evaluated, the project workers had gathered enough information from projects and candidate feedback to begin to draw some conclusions about what makes for success in running joint programmes. As in previous studies (Jones, 1986), the importance of having a balance of the different professionals in the group was stressed. Where this had not been possible in some of the pilots, participants who were in a minority had felt overwhelmed or marginalised.

Project workers found that participants on joint programmes needed time at the beginning to get to know each other and each other's roles. Where this did not happen, participants seemed to want more sessions in uni-professional groups and failed to see the benefit of shared learning. A lecture approach where theory was presented formally was not successful on the joint programmes. A workshop or problem-centred approach worked a great deal better.

The overall conclusion of the project workers was that the initiative had been successful and well-received, but that it would need to adapt considerably in order to adjust to the further wave of changes in service and education delivery. These changes, which are outlined in the next section, resulted in the project workers being inundated with requests for advice or consultancy about the potential for establishing a range of related interprofessional initiatives.

THE NEW WAVE OF CHANGES

Between 1993 and 1995, the changes in service delivery and higher education institutions and a number of government imperatives

144

meant that interprofessional education and training moved steadily up the agenda. The project manager and the development workers noticed the way in which JPTI changed from being a somewhat marginal initiative to one on which speakers were regularly asked for at conferences, and requests for literature came from all over the UK.

Service delivery

By 1993, the implementation of the Community Care Act was well bedded in, and nurses and occupational therapists were being appointed as care managers along with social workers and people holding Care Awards at S/NVQ level 3. Chronic problems of communication between social services and GPs were brought to a head when GPs complained that they were not being consulted or informed about local community care plans. Social workers and care managers complained that GPs were refusing to play their part in assessment and care packaging (Hudson, 1994).

Problems about collaboration between health and social services were also emerging because of the eagerness of Trust Hospitals to reduce waiting lists and free beds by discharging patients into the community, once treatment was complete. The care in the community of people with mental health problems was another major concern leading to demands for improved collaboration and better interprofessional education and training.

While interprofessional training around child protection had become well-established in the late eighties, additional needs for interprofessional collaboration with regard to children were being identified. Local authorities and health authorities were being asked to draw up joint plans for children along the lines of their joint community care plans. The focus was to be on children in need. Research indicated that children who were being accommodated by local authorities were likely to have both their health and their education badly neglected, again emphasising the urgency for better collaboration between professionals.

Changes in management and delivery of professional education

Meanwhile nursing schools and other pre-registration health courses were being relocated in university faculties, side by side with schools of social work. The need for economy and efficiency, apart from anything else, led the managers of these new large departments to seek opportunities for shared learning.

Further major changes following the publication of the Functions and Manpower Review of the NHS (NHS, 1994) were being anticipated by managers, education providers and professional bodies and were leading to increased interest in interprofessional education. The shifts, which were confirmed in a letter from the National Health Service Executive (Jarrold, 1995), will mean:

- the abolition (by 1996) of Regional Health Authorities and reorganisation of the NHS Executive with eight Regional Offices;
- that workforce planning and determining intake levels to education and training programmes will become primarily an employer responsibility;
- that purchasers, NHS health care providers, GPs, social services authorities, the voluntary and private sectors, will join together in consortia to determine the level of student intakes. Consortia will take over the responsibility for holding budgets and contracting with education providers.

The letter encourages consortia to engage in 'local development activity around, for example multi-professional education or management development'.

Another body, the Higher Education Quality Council (HEQC) which was established following the 1992 Further and Higher Education Act, has also been active in linking the NHS providers, the education providers and the professional bodies to encourage the development of a common approach to quality standards for the education and training of health care professionals.

Development of national occupational standards

The Care Sector Consortium, which is the lead body established by the Employment Department to develop national standards for care, commissioned consultants to produce a functional map of the entire health and care sector. The purpose was to develop occupational standards for the sector and to identify gaps or overlaps in existing educational provision.

Some professional bodies expressed doubts which were shared by many educationalists in institutes of higher education (Smithers and Robinson, 1993); these focused on the government's perceived

146

intention that employers, rather than professionals or educationalists, should take over the establishment of standards. Barr (1995)
found that professionals were worried that:

> 'at para-professional levels, demarcations between occupations
> are being redrawn and crossed and may conceivably be removed
> . . . as common transferable competences are established . . .
> Will this lead to the emergence of community carers as a new
> unified occupation in place of numerous other para-professions?
> Alternatively, is this the beginning of the decomposition of
> occupational groups as such, individual workers being contracted
> in future not by role or by job title but by a particular constella-
> tion of competences.'
> (Barr, 1994)

In a survey of professional bodies undertaken by the HEQC:

> 'A majority of the professional bodies expressed uncertainty over
> their relationship with NCVQ and concern over the likely impact
> of S/NVQs. In some cases "hostility" would not be too strong a
> description of their reaction.'
> (Brown, R., 1994)

Social work led the way on professional standards development
when, in 1994, CCETSW agreed to work with the Care Sector
Consortium to develop occupational standards for social workers.
The requirements for the new Dip. SW which the Government
decreed should be implemented from October 1995, were to be
derived from these occupational standards. The agreement secured
by CCETSW was that while the content and the assessment criteria
of Dip. SW would be informed by the occupational standards, they
would remain entirely under the control of CCETSW. Dip. SW
would continue to be the only recognised social work qualification
and would be delivered at a minimum of Dip. HE level.

In the meantime, the Care Sector Consortium expressed its
intention to develop national occupational standards for three
interlinked areas of health care – complementary medicine, health
promotion and seven professions allied to medicine. The Health and
Care Professions' Education Forum proposed to the Care Sector
Consortium the idea of a feasibility study to identify Standards in
Common at the point of exit from Higher Education and entry into
practice. The Health Education Authority and a small group of

complementary health professions put forward their own projects and the three groups agreed to work jointly at appropriate points and levels.

The development work for the project was to be UK-wide, involving representatives of the practitioner groups who work in the NHS, local authorities (including criminal justice), the private sector, the voluntary sector, education and training and industry. The project aimed to examine 'areas of common registration practice' which were defined as 'common to two or more of the professional groups concerned, i.e. which are not unique to one professional group.' The brief also included an evaluation of existing national occupational standards for their relevance to the groups concerned in anticipation that overlaps would be identified which might have implications for job boundaries and/or shared learning.

Just as this project began to get under way, the long awaited Vision Paper on the development of vocational qualifications to levels 4 and 5 (Department of Employment, 1995) was published. In Annex 1 an extract from a letter from the Secretary of State for Employment is used to explain government policy:

'It will be important . . . to consider in due course how GNVQs and NVQs can fit together coherently with academic and professional qualifications to ensure effective progression to full occupational competence at work which takes full account of the interests of Higher Education.'
(Department of Employment, 1994)

The paper itself guarantees full involvement of professional and statutory bodies and of higher education institutions in determining,

'the nature of qualifications appropriate for different sectors and on the relationships between them. In particular areas of possible credit accumulation and transfer would be identified and mechanisms agreed to allow ready articulation between them'.

Although this paper had been anticipated for some time, it is important to note that at this stage there was no commitment by any of the professions involved in standards development to develop NVQs at levels 4 and 5 as replacements for, or equivalents to professional qualifications.

Attitudes to shared learning at qualifying/pre-registration level

The debate about the best stage at which to begin shared learning had been a continuous theme throughout the life of the JPTI, and there was a noticeable attitudinal shift between 1993 and 1995. Interprofessional training at post-qualifying level raised little controversy, and interprofessional Masters programmes and 'top-up' degrees mushroomed during the period of JPTI. However, there was initially considerable resistance to the notion of shared learning at the pre-registration stage. The pioneers in this respect were joint programmes for nurses and social workers preparing to work with people with learning disabilities (Brown, J., 1994). Following the validation of two Dip. SW/Project 2000 programmes in 1991, the ENB put a moratorium on the development of further programmes of this kind.

It is significant that in 1994 this moratorium was lifted. When this happened a surprising number of programmes immediately expressed their interest in gaining joint validation and were also interested in JPTI. Also in 1994, a report by the Department of Health into occupational therapy services in social services departments (SSI, 1994) recommended joint training of social workers and occupational therapists at qualifying level. Colleagues from CCETSW and the COT who had collaborated on the steering group of JPTI established a feasibility study in response to the report. In an even more radical move CCETSW and the Social Services Inspectorate jointly sponsored a project with the Centre for Advancement of Inter Professional Education to explore the potential for joint training between doctors and social workers (CAIPE, 1996; Vanclay, 1996).

Developments in training of practice teachers

Meanwhile, the training of practice teachers in all three professions was being reviewed between 1993 and 1996. In social work (CCETSW, 1995) and occupational therapy (COT, 1994) an outcomes approach which described the knowledge, values and skills that a competent practice teacher/clinical supervisor would be expected to display replaced the previous prescribed curriculum. Similarly, in their document on standards for post-registration practice, the UKCC (1994) described under the heading of clinical practice leadership that candidates will 'ensure effective learning experiences and opportunity to achieve learning outcomes for students through preceptorship, mentorship, counselling, clinical supervision and provision of an educational environment.'

The product of the review of Community Practice Teacher (CPT) programmes is likely to be a more flexible and outcome-oriented approach which will adapt well for sharing with other professions (Langlands, 1995).

In all three professions the resources, both in terms of workload relief and finance for releasing professionals to attend long courses, were increasingly drying up. In social work and occupational therapy this led to the development of models of training by which candidates might learn and develop in the workplace and demonstrate their competence via portfolio assessment. Both professions were interested in the potential for articulation with the NVQs offered by the Training and Development Lead Body (TDLB) now Employment Occupational Standards Council.

In many parts of the country, CPT programmes were closing down or running less frequently through lack of sponsored candidates. Purchasers were reluctant to send community nurses on practice teacher programmes, partly because the qualification entitled the successful candidate to an enhanced salary, and partly because Project 2000 meant that there were fewer candidates on community nursing courses. As profession-specific CPT courses became less viable, the nurses expressed a growing interest in joint courses.

LOOKING TO THE FUTURE

In March 1995, JPTI held its final conference. This was well-attended by an enthusiastic network of professionals which went well beyond the original JPTI project participants and the steering group. While the main mission of JPTI had always been an improved service for users, there had, until now, been a marked absence of user-participation in the project. The strong and effective user-presence at the final conference was very supportive of interprofessional collaboration, on condition that users and carers were treated as equal partners in the alliance.

The occupational therapy officer from the Department of Health gave an encouraging keynote address in which she stressed that joint training and shared learning were a means of enriching and improving professional training, not a way of diminishing it or watering it down (Vanclay, 1995). She reminded the conference that the analyses of complaints and Ombudsman's enquiries continue to indicate that breakdowns in communication between agencies are still causing major distress to consumers. She paid tribute to the champions of change 'who have been breaking new ground; trying to change attitudes; challenging the stereotypes and cost comfortable conventions . . .', and she acknowledged 'the gains and richness of creativity and exploration' which had been demonstrated in the development of JPTI.

In addition to the two workshops run by service users, sessions were organised on the following topics:

- The development of shared learning between General Practitioners and other health professionals;
- The best way to approach gaining validation by more than one body;
- Effective evaluation and promotion strategies;
- The assessment and accreditation of practice in the workplace at post qualifying level;
- How to tackle issues of culture and values when running interprofessional programmes;
- How to gain management support and commitment to joint training initiatives.

Participants agreed to build on the networks established through JPTI and to utilise the Newsletter of the Centre for the Advancement of Inter Professional Education to publicise progress and developments. The JPTI development workers stressed the need for newly developing initiatives between nurses and social workers, occupational therapists and social workers, GPs and other professionals to incorporate a joint practice teaching component in their plans. ENB, COT and CCETSW undertook to review the core module with a view to updating it and making it more relevant to the new context of training for health and care professionals.

CONCLUSION

While JPTI was undoubtedly successful in terms of generating interest and enthusiasm for joint training, influencing attitudes and contributing to the development of a growing interprofessional network, it was less successful in its specific aim which was to establish joint practice teaching courses for nurses, social workers and occupational therapists.

This very much bears out the view of Dr R. Jones (1986), one of the early pioneers of joint training, who said that:

'multi-disciplinary training is almost universally supported and almost invariably not practised'.

JPTI's limited success relied to a large degree on the availability of pump-priming grants or the enthusiasm of individual project leaders. Of the 12 projects involved overall, only three are likely to continue as mainstream programmes at the time of writing. On the other hand, CCETSW, ENB and COT are receiving numerous enquiries from people interested in establishing new joint programmes. Growing pressures on staff and the costing of their time by managers mean that unless joint training projects become part of the main stream, they are unlikely to survive their champions or their pump-priming money.

The JPTI research showed that the commitment and involvement of managers and purchasers was a crucial success factor. It also indicated that managers were keen on improved collaboration and were less concerned about preserving professional boundaries than were practitioners and educationalists. It will be interesting to see whether, when employers have an even firmer hold on the purse strings with the new consortia arrangements, this will influence the position.

At the final JPTI conference, participants were very aware that although there had been significant change and progress on the interprofessional front since the launching conference in 1990, the underlying fears and suspicions expressed then had in no way been diminished. In the words of Sheelagh Richards, Occupational Therapy Officer at DH and the keynote speaker at the conference, this constituted 'an underlying concern that interprofessional or multi-professional education was an alternative respectable language for deskilling', or, in the words of one of the JPTI study respondents when asked about the government's purpose in promoting joint training, 'They have lost our trust. We need to trust that their motives really are patient care and not just economic.'

Perceived attacks on the professionals, for example the 1995 nurses' pay offer and insistence on local negotiations, the government-initiated media attack on social work values and the removal of the training of probation officers from Higher Education, may make the professions even more defensive and increase the siege mentality and resistance to interprofessional education.

On the other hand, if the juggernaut of occupational standards development is widely embraced by employers, and if in their role as planners and purchasers of education they see NVQs as an efficient and cost-effective way forward, the professions may have no alternative but to collaborate in the proposals for levels 4 and 5 as described in the Vision Paper.

If the latter scenario prevails, the drawing of the functional map by the CSC may result in the outcome described by Thompson and Mathias (1992), who suggest that the competence approach to professional education is likely to lead to the identification of competences which are the same for each profession:

'When this has been achieved, it will be possible to think again about the structuring and organising of professions and occupations within the helping services. If the balance is found to be weighted more heavily towards shared competence, perhaps a common stem or occupation with many branches or specialisms, might be the best way to reorganise the helping professions.'

This approach has already been adopted in a very positive way in a pilot programme called Education for Holistic Care in Finland. (Lämsa et al., 1994). The programme is committed to the notion that because health, welfare, production and the environment are so closely interlinked, the training of professionals for those fields should also be integrated. The organisers of the programme believe that 'the structure of the working community is changing as hierarchies collapse and organisational levels disappear. In future, social and health work will be organised as a holistic exercise between different fields'.

Participants in the JPTI project, along with other health and welfare professionals and educationalists would almost certainly subscribe to this ideal. However, further convincing is required that the means proposed for achieving it really is directed towards improved patient care and not towards a cheaper service run by staff who are trained to perform specific tasks but not to question or to critically evaluate the service they are offering.

References

Barr, H. (1994) *Perspectives on Shared Learning*. London: Council for the Advancement of Interprofessional Education in Primary Care.

Bartholomew, A. Davis, J. and Weinstein, J. (1995) Final Report to the Steering Group on the Join Practice Teaching Initiative. Central Council for Education and Training in Social Work, CCETSW (Unpublished).

Bartholomew, A., Davis, J. and Weinstein, J. (1996) *Interprofessional Education and Training – Developing New Models*. Report of the Joint Practice Teaching Initiative 1990-1995. London: CCETSW.

Brown, J. (1994) The Hybrid Worker – Lessons based upon a study of employers involved with two pioneer joint qualifying training courses. University of York.

Brown, R. (1994) Quality and standards: The HEQC Perspective, reported in Quality in Higher Education Project (1995) *Proceedings of the Third QHE Seminar: Quality and Standards – The Role of the Professions*. Birmingham: QHE.

Brown, S. (1993) *Practice Makes Perfect: A Review of Issues and Lessons from the Joint Practice Teaching Initiative*. CCETSW.

CAIPE (1996) *A Report for Social Work Educators: Developing Shared Learning with Medical Students and General Practitioners*. London: CCETSW.

Central Council for Education and Training in Social Work (1989) *Improving Standards in Practice Learning: Requirements and Guidance for the Approval of Agencies and the Accreditation and Training of Practice Teachers*. Paper 26.3 London: CCETSW.

Central Council for Education and Training in Social Work (1990) Conference Report: Joint Training of Practice Teachers, York. London: CCETSW (unpublished).

Central Council for Education and Training in Social Work (1991) Joint Training of Practice Teachers; Report of the Workshop for Funded Projects. London: CCETSW (unpublished).

Central Council for Education and Training in Social Work (1995a) *Assuring Quality, in the Diploma in Social Work – Rules and Requirements for the Dip. SW*. London: CCETSW.

Central Council for Education and Training in Social Work (1995b) *Rules and Requirements for Practice Teaching Programmes*. London: CCETSW.

College of Occupational Therapists (1988) *Post-Registration Studies Committee. Adopting the Sequential Approach to Clinical Education.* London: COT.

College of Occupational Therapists (1994) *Recommended Requirements for the Accreditation of Fieldwork Educators.* London: COT.

Department of Employment (1995) *A Vision for Higher Level Vocational Qualifications.* London: HMSO.

Department of Health (DH) (1989a) *Working for Patients.* Working paper 10: Education and Training. London: HMSO.

Department of Health (DH) (1989b) *Caring for People.* Cm 849, London: HMSO.

Ellis, R. (1988) *Professional Competence and Quality Assurance in the Caring Professions.* London: Chapman & Hall.

English National Board (ENB) for Nursing, Midwifery and Health Visiting (1991) *Guidelines for the Community Practice Teacher Course.* Circular 1991/21/MB. London: ENB.

Hayek, F. A. (1960) The Constitution of Liberty. London: Routledge and Kegan Paul.

Hevey, D. (1992) The potential of National Vocational Qualifications to make multidisciplinary training a reality. *Journal of Interprofessional Care*, 6(3) pp. 215–21. Carfax Publishing, Oxfordshire.

Home Office, Department of Health, Department of Education and Science, Welsh Office (1991) *Working Together Under The Children Act 1989.* London: HMSO.

Hudson, B. (1994) 'Breaks in the Chain' *Health Service Journal*, 105(5399) pp. 24–6.

Hunter, D. and Wistow, G. (1987) *Community Care in Britain – Variations on a Theme.* London: King's Fund.

Illich, I. (1977) *Disabling Professions.* London: Marion Boyars.

Jarrold, K. (1995) *Education and Training in the New NHS.* Letter ref. EL(95)28. London: National Health Services Executive.

Johnson, T. (1972) *Professions and Power.* London: Macmillan.

Jones, R. V. H. (1986) *Working Together – Learning Together.* Occasional paper 33. London: Royal College of General Practitioners.

Lämsa, A., Hietanen, I., and Lämsa, J. (1994) Education for Holistic Care: A Pilot Programme in Finland. *Journal of Interprofessional Care*, 8(1) pp. 31–43, Carfax Publishing, Oxfordshire.

155

Langlands, T. (1995) Personal communication.

Lincoln, Y. S. (1985) *Organisational Theory and Enquiry. The Paradigm Revolution.* London: Sage.

Minford, P. (1987) 'The Role of the Social Services: A View from the New Right' in Loney, M., Babcock, B., Clark J., Cochrane, A., Graham, P. and Wilson, M. (eds), *The State or the Market.* London: Sage.

National Health Service (1994) *Functions and Manpower Review of the NHS.* London: HMSO.

Reason, P. and Rowan, J. (eds) (1981) *Human Enquiry – A Sourcebook of New Paradigm Research.* Chichester: John Wiley.

Smithers, A. and Robinson, P. (1993) *Changing Colleges: Further Education in the Market Place.* London: Council for Industry and Higher Education.

SSI (1994) *Occupational Therapy – The Community Contribution.* Report on Local Authority Occupational Therapy Services. London: HMSO.

Thompson, T. and Mathias, P. eds (1992) *Standards and Mental Handicap: Keys to Competence.* London: Baillière Tindall.

United Kingdom Central Council for Nursing, Midwifery and Health Visiting (1994) *The Council's Standards for Education and Practice Following Registration.* Registrar's letter 20/1994. London: UKCC.

Vanclay, L. (1995) Report of the Final Conference of JPTI – Coventry March, 1995. London: CCETSW.

Vanclay, L. (1996) *Sustaining Collaboration between General Practitioners and Social Workers.* London: CAIPE.

Walton, I. (1989) Workforce Needs and Training Resources. The development of the first ENB/CCETSW validated joint training courses in mental handicap. University of York, Dept. of Social Policy (unpublished).

Webb, D. (1992) 'Competences, Contracts and Cadres: Common Themes in the Social Control of Nurse and Social Work Education'. *Journal of Interprofessional Care*, 6(3), pp. 223–30. Carfax Publishing, Oxfordshire.

Weinstein, J. (1993) 'What are the barriers to implementing successful interprofessional training programmes in the context of the mixed economy and the changing roles and relationships of the caring professions? An action research study of the Joint Practice Teaching Initiative (JPTI).' M.Sc. Dissertation, South Bank University, London.

CHAPTER EIGHT

The Functional Map of Health and Social Care[*]

Lindsay Mitchell and Margaret Coats

This chapter looks at issues of interprofessional working through taking the perspective of the functional map of health and social care. The functional map is an attempt to provide an overview of all the work roles in the sector in an integrated and coherent way. It does this by looking at how those who work in the sector aim to meet the needs of service users, whatever their professional background and training and however this is carried out, by a single profession or through interprofessional work.

The chapter is divided into the following sections:

1. The purpose of a functional map – why develop it, what is it for?
2. The development processes used to produce the functional map – who helped to develop it and how?
3. The ideas and approaches which underpin the map – how is the work of the sector described?

[*]This chapter draws from the work of the Care Sector Consortium's Functional Mapping Project for Health and Social Care. The two authors were closely involved with that project. Lindsay Mitchell was project director of the team of consultants from Prime R&D Ltd which undertook the research and development work. Margaret Coats is the director of the CSC and was responsible for overseeing the progress of the project and now for ensuring that the functional map is used to its optimum value in the ongoing work of the Consortium. Both authors wish to acknowledge the huge debt to the considerable number of individuals and organisations in the sector who made valuable contributions to the work, members of the Consortium who guided the progress of the project, and to Tom Caple and Jackie Sturton, colleagues at Prime who formed the project team.

4. The potential uses of the map – what can we do with it now that we have it?
5. The next stages in the development and use of the map – what next?

THE PURPOSE OF A FUNCTIONAL MAP

A functional map presents a holistic view of the outcomes expected of work roles in a particular sector. A functional map has several features which make it different from other ways of describing work. It:

- describes intended results or outcomes of work – not job titles, activities, tasks or skills;
- is based on agreed best practice;
- is forward-looking rather than reflective;
- explicitly reflects underpinning values and ethics.

A map is a description of occupational competence. Competence is defined as the achievement of outcomes associated with particular work roles. Statements within a map describe the fundamental nature of work roles in a sector. A work role, in this context, is not a job (such as occupational therapy manager) nor a set of tasks, nor an organisational rank (such as senior social worker) nor a professional role descriptor (such as health visitor, probation officer, psychiatrist, physiological measurement technician or operating department practitioner). The map makes no specific reference to particular occupational groups. Some will 'find' their functions in one part of the map alone; others will be able to identify their roles across a number of different parts of the map which, taken together, will describe their particular job.

The main purpose of developing a functional map is to provide a comprehensive and coherent framework for developing national occupational standards and National Vocational Qualifications (NVQs) (or in Scotland Scottish Vocational Qualifications – SVQs). Nationally, the responsibility for developing functional maps lies with Occupational Standards Councils or Lead Bodies, which are groupings of employment interests for different sectors, recognised by the Department for Education and Employment. (Occupational Standards Councils are essentially large lead bodies which have the responsibility for developing standards and NVQs/SVQs across whole or larger sectors than do lead bodies.)

The Occupational Standards Council for the care sector is the Care Sector Consortium which is formed from representatives from employers, employees, professional groups and education and training interests across the four UK countries of England, Northern Ireland, Scotland and Wales. The Care Sector Consortium's remit includes those who both purchase and provide health care services, social care services and criminal justice services in the statutory, private and voluntary sectors across the four UK countries. A simplified picture showing the main employers is shown in Figure 8.1.

	Health Care Services	Social Care Services (including Child Care and Education and Community Work)	Criminal Justice Services
Statutory Sector	NHS (Eng. Scot, Wales)	Local authority Social Service/Social Work Departments (Eng., Scot., Wales)	Probation Services + SSDs (E,W) Probation Board for NI + HSSBs (NI)
	Health & Social Services Boards (NI)		Social Work Departments (Scot)
Voluntary Sector	Large number of voluntary sector organisations across all services		
Private Sector	Large number of private sector organisations + private practitioners – predominantly providing health care services		Very small number of private sector organisations

Figure 8.1 The care sector's main employers

Whilst it is not possible to provide an accurate figure of the sector's total workforce, Table 8.1 summarises the data presented in this chapter. These figures mean, in effect, that the approximate size of the care sector workforce in 1993 was 1 885 820. This figure should be taken as an underestimate of the true number of individuals employed as no data was available for independent hospitals or other independent practitioners; much of the data is given in Whole Time Equivalent posts which understates the number of individuals employed; and estimates for the voluntary sector vary so widely that they have not been included. It is probably, therefore, safe to say that there are over two million

Statutory Sector	NHS (UK, WTE)	1 053 250
	Social Services (UK, WTE)	291 600
	Probation (Eng. number)*	16 200
Voluntary Sector	between 50 000 and 250 000 across the UK	
Private Sector	Nursing and residential homes (Eng + Wales, WTE)	403 900 no data
	Independent hospitals	59 000
	General dental practitioners/auxiliaries (Eng + Scot, number)*	11 080 20 790
	High street opticians etc (UK?)	over 30 000
	Community pharmacists (GB, number)*	no data
	Alternative/complementary medicine practitioners (UK?, number)	
	Other independent practitioners	

* Most of the data are expressed in WTE (Whole Time Equivalents) except for those marked * for which the number of people is known but not whether they are whole-time or part-time.

individuals employed within the sector with many more offering their services in voluntary or informal carer roles.

The sector is consequently of enormous numerical size and includes a wide diversity of roles and functions. This not only provided a real challenge in the development of the functional map but is also an issue for those who work within the sector itself as they seek to conceptualise their role. At the outset of the project it was necessary to develop a comprehensive consultation framework of all those who had a rightful say in the development of the functional map. A structure for the framework was developed which identified the scope and nature of interests which should be included and information on relevant organisations was sought from sources throughout the project, as more organisations heard about the work and expressed an interest in being involved. By the end of the project over 300 organisations were included in the framework.

Occupational standards are developed by occupations within different sectors identifying the nature and quality of competence people need in the work environment – the expectations of different work roles. These expectations are expressed in a commonly-agreed format of units of competence, elements of competence, their associated performance criteria and statement of range. The title of an element of competence describes an occupational outcome – what people are expected to achieve. The performance criteria describe critical performance indicators and are, as such, benchmark descriptions – how you would know that someone can do what is described in the element title. The range statements describe the circumstances or contexts to which the element of competence and its associated performance criteria apply. The element of competence, its associated performance criteria and statement of range together are an occupational standard. Units of competence are groupings of elements of competence and are used as the basis for structuring National (or Scottish) Vocational Qualifications. Occupational standards are developed into vocational qualifications by selecting groups of units which are relevant to particular work roles, and attaching to them an assessment process by which an individual's achievement of the standards can be validly and reliably assessed. The complete qualification, or a suite of qualifications (that is a group(s) of standards plus the assessment process), is submitted to the National Council for Vocational Qualifications (NCVQ) or the Scottish Vocational Education Council (SCOTVEC in Scotland). The qualifications are evaluated by these bodies against a set of criteria (the NVQ/SVQ criteria and guidance) and if they are of sufficient quality they are recognised as an NVQ/SVQ and acknowledged as such. NCVQ does not award NVQs itself, this is done through a number of awarding bodies each of whom have to meet the criteria for submission of the qualification before they can be accredited.

However, the map is not:

- *a set of standards* – it provides a starting point for standards development. Selecting the starting point for all standards projects, whether current or new, thus becomes an important issue when the map is used in the future;
- *a qualifications framework* – in the past, the CSC has sometimes published its standards in the form of qualifications frameworks (units grouped into qualifications at different S/NVQ levels), and it appears that these may have shaped expectations of what a 'map' is or does. One potential problem is that qualifications have levels attached to them (either explicitly or implicitly) which a functional map does not and there is the possibility that people

161

will attempt to identify 'levels' within the map. The map describes only functions, and functions in broad terms (not even as units of competence). It has nothing to say about level, which is an issue for qualification design and which arises only when standards have been developed and grouped;

- *an organisational framework* – the map does not present a picture of how care is currently organised in the sector, who should take responsibility for what, or the value in terms of payment which should be associated with each of the functions. The map describes only the functions in the sector, it does not say who should undertake them or what their relative value is.

A functional map is the product of an analysis, and consequently the final product should conform with the usual rules of analysis.

- All of the data should be classified systematically, so that there are logical relationships between the components of the map and no duplication of function within the map.
- The analysis is 'top down' proceeding from the general to the specific – in the case of a functional map, derived through functional analysis, the 'top' is represented by the *key purpose statement*.
- The key purpose is a 'definition' of the entire occupational area in outcome terms and it should be capable of describing the occupational sector, organisations which operate specifically within the sector, key groups or departments in organisations, as well as the expectations of individuals. This is a strength of the analysis since it provides broad links between individual performance and national standards. The development of the key purpose is an important stage in the analysis because it is from this statement that all other stages are developed.
- At each of the later stages of analysis it is important to decide the 'rule' which should be applied – and the rule should ensure that the components follow general classification rules:

  - it continues to be a complete description of the occupation;
  - it generates categories which are exclusive;
  - it is a credible reflection of what happens in the occupation.

Many different rules could be used to classify an occupation. So it is important to choose rules which make most sense within the sector – which represent practice most accurately, which are likely to be credible to employers, practitioners and educators

As the map must be credible with those who are to use it or may be affected by it, it is developed through working with 'key' groups/ organisations who have a direct interest in the performance of the work roles – either because the group is representative of people who fill the work role, employs those who fill the work role, regulates those who practise, or educates and trains them. This does not, of course, give everyone involved in the development of a map a licence to comment on and shape every work role within it. Depending on the scope of a map, it will reflect the expectations of different groups/organisations in respect of different work roles. Key groups and organisations may, of course, differ in their expectations. The map must take account of significant differences in expectations.

Functional maps tell us nothing of how a sector is organised, who performs which role or how many perform a particular role, nor does it tell us about the current qualifications and development which are used by individuals and organisations in the sector. There are a number of features of a functional map which need to be emphasised in its use:

1. *A functional map describes broad functions but does not say how these functions are to be organised*
   Whilst the map describes what has to be achieved within health and social care, it is neutral about how and by whom these expectations are to be fulfilled. A map says nothing about how expectations are translated into activities, tasks and jobs, whether they are carried out at particular levels within an organisational or social hierarchy, whether they are associated with one professional group or many, how many people work in the sector, how they are trained and employed, or how they move from one work role to another. It describes functions but does not allocate them to groups of people, determine how human resources are developed or how people are allocated to jobs in order to achieve these standards. These, and other related decisions, such as the level of investment in human resources, may be informed, but are not pre-determined by, the structure and content of the map.

2. *A functional map is a new way of describing health and social care*
   The functional map brings all of the work roles within the sector into one framework, describing their interrelationship in a consistent and coherent way. This may be seen as a new way of describing health and social care which some respondents in

the consultation described as 'enlightening' and the debate engendered by the consultation was reported as 'one of the best foci for staff development for many years'. However, this same novelty may be a barrier to the effective use of the map. Understanding what it describes, and the nature and degree of abstraction of its statements, is essential for its proper use and its credibility. This in turn means that people are likely to need considerable help to understand the map before it is used.

3. *The functional map is only one way of describing the sector*
Whilst the functional map is a novel way of describing the sector which individuals may find exciting, it presents information of one kind only. It describes general expectations of what people should be able to do. The map does not present priorities for further work nor does it make decisions for organisations. In short, the functional map provides one kind of information; it is not a 'magic rabbit' which answers all known problems! Another key challenge for the CSC in its own work and in promoting the use of the map to others, is in enabling users to understand what the map is able to do and what it is not.

DEVELOPMENT PROCESS

The functional map was developed through a project undertaken in three main phases from June 1993–July 1994:

Phase 1   Development of the consultation framework for the map; Initial development of the functional map via desk research and mapping workshops.

Phase 2   Verification and further development of the functional map via postal consultation.

Phase 3   Development of proposals for linking the functional map to other related initiatives.

A first draft of the map was developed from analysing information from the field and making initial proposals as to the content and structure of the map. From those first proposals, the map was continually developed and redrafted on a consultative basis working with representatives from the different parts of the sector. In the first instance, the map was taken out to workshops comprised of practitioners from across the whole of health and social care who were asked to examine the first drafts and make suggestions as to how it might be improved. Following redrafting a national consultation took place where representative organisations were briefed about the purpose and nature of the map and how they might best consult on it. The map was then issued to key named representatives of those organisations for them to organise their own consultation as they best thought fit. Following feedback the map was once more redrafted and taken to workshops of representatives of organisations for them to consider its contents and the implications of its development.

Identifying and contacting appropriate occupations to be involved in the workshops was a major undertaking, given the size and scope of the sector. In particular, the number of different occupations and professions which could have been involved on the health care side was potentially huge. A number of key groups in health care had also had little previous contact with the work of the CSC and there were therefore no established routes of access to them. This was in contrast to the social care side where there are fewer professional groups and where the main organisations (such as professional bodies, employer organisations and trade unions) had long-standing links with the Consortium and its work.

In order to address this dual challenge of firstly identifying and contacting a representative sample of health care occupations, and secondly accommodating them within the workshop programme, two measures were taken by the project.

Firstly, given the larger number of occupations in health care it was decided to devote four of the events to health care and two to social care. Whilst 'integrated' workshops which mixed practitioners from different parts of the health and social care spectrum might have better reflected the aim of producing an integrated map of the sector, it would have been extremely difficult to organise appropriate representation at such events.

Secondly, a regional health authority agreed to draw up a 'sample frame' which identified a representative range of occupations and professions to involve, and then to identify and contact, appropriate people within the region to fill the workshop places. The sample frame attempted to include as many roles and functions as possible within the limited number of places available (30 per workshop). The four workshops were each given a different focus to cover the different contexts and settings within which health care is delivered. The major organisational split in the NHS between community, acute, and primary care gave the focus to three of the workshops with the fourth concentrating on purchaser and educational roles. A very different approach was taken to organising the social care workshops. Rather than having a regional focus, they were organised on a national basis with representative national organisations (such as professional bodies and employer organisations) being asked to nominate practitioners to attend. In the workshops, discussions were mainly carried out in pairs or small groups, with participants recording their comments on cards which were, when time allowed, posted up on the wall so that ideas could be shared amongst the whole group.

An exercise like this will never be representative in any statistical sense as it is based on interpretation of qualitative data. The functional map in its current form describes what is expected of different roles, as described (and subsequently confirmed, amended or modified) by participants in each of the three phases of the project. By definition the map describes what is considered to be best practice from the different perspectives of the many individuals and organisations who have contributed to its creation. Moreover, the process of describing functions is, as the project process illustrates, iterative. Should the Consortium seek further views on the map, these will in turn influence the way expectations are described. The map then is not a statistical representation of what good practice is, but a mirror reflecting the (informed and experienced) views of the project participants. The 'representativeness' of the map is in the relationship between its statements and good practice on the ground, as described by those who are experts in the different functions.

This means that while it was important to offer every possible group the opportunity to contribute, the development of the map could not be halted by those who chose not to, or were unable to, participate during its development phase. This does not invalidate the map, but it does mean that some important 'reflections' will not be as clearly evidenced as they might be. The map is as accurate as the data available allowed. It reflects the input and feedback received from a wide range of individuals and organisations in the sector and provides a basis for moving forward. However, it is not fixed for all time and remains open to challenge and further development – in fact this is what the Consortium intends – to review the content and structure of the map as it is used in its development work. As the map is constructed through a process of debate, discussion and negotiation, it is socially constructed and not a physical phenomenon in its own right. The social construction cannot only change as the sector changes over time, it should change and must change to better reflect new challenges, new technologies, new ways of improving services to users and so on. If the map fails to retain its focus on the future, it will have outlived its usefulness.

IDEAS AND APPROACHES WHICH UNDERPIN THE MAP

There are a number of key ideas and approaches on which the map is based and these have affected the key purpose statement of the sector – the starting point for the analysis of the map – and all its subsequent content and structure. The key purpose statement is critical simply because everything else is derived from it. The debate on issues and approaches centred around:

- the key concepts within the key purpose and hence within the functional map;
- the comprehensiveness of the key purpose statement as a representative description of the sector as a whole – this is linked to those groups and roles which are, and are not, included in the domain of the health and social care sector.

The first draft, in July 1993, was:

'Enable and empower individuals, families and communities to achieve their optimum health and well being.'

By November 1993 it had been modified and this draft was used in the consultative workshops in January 1994:

'Enable individuals, families and communities to optimise their health and social well being.'

The draft that was used for the postal consultation (February 1994) was:

'Enable the population to enhance and maintain its health and social well being, balancing the needs of individuals, communities and society.'

As a result of the feedback from the consultation, the final statement of key purpose is:

'Enable individuals, families, groups and communities to optimise their health and social well-being, balancing their respective needs with those of wider society and the available resources'.

These changes in the key purpose reflect the debate engendered by the project over the key concepts within the map.

The beneficiaries of the sector

The original analysis identified individuals, families and communities. During the initial workshops, the term 'families' caused problems as it was identified with a government push on 'back to basics' – families being seen as a husband, a wife and their two children. In short, the use of the term 'families' was seen to be supporting a moral crusade with which a number of individuals were unhappy. In the consultation edition, the term 'communities' was adopted as a global term to mean communities of relationship, of interest and of geography. This was felt by many to be too broad to cover the immediate social group, which may itself be the direct beneficiary of 'care'. The omnibus term used in the consultation draft of 'population' was also seen as far too inexact, or too partial, having meaning only in the context of large-scale planning or in particular areas, such as epidemiology. In short, there is, it appears, no neat way of defining the sector's beneficiaries. Those who work in the sector appear happiest with the phrase '*individuals, families, groups and communities*' as this best identifies the range of work which may be undertaken and the inter-relationship between the different parts. The term 'population' has been retained in those areas of the map to which it specifically applies (such as in the examples given above).

The objective of the sector

The phrase 'health and social well-being' has been accepted throughout the development of the map and there has been no question that it lies at the heart of the sector. It has been used throughout the development of the functional map to encompass all aspects of social, physical, intellectual, communication and emotional/psychological 'health' including the notion of 'being at one with oneself'. The term does not signify that a particular view of 'health and social well-being' is being promoted but recognises that different groups may use different concepts. The focus has been very clearly on 'health and social well-being' in contrast to problem-oriented/illness models.

The term 'optimise' was used originally linked to 'health and social well-being' but was rejected with vehemence in the Phase 1 workshops. This appeared to be because:

- people confused the term 'optimise' with 'maximise' and therefore assumed that it was suggested that everyone could achieve the maximum possible health – inappropriate for the terminally ill and many others;
- it was interpreted as 'making the best of what you have got', and by inference 'making do' with inadequate resources.

In the consultation draft, the clause 'enhance and maintain' was used in an attempt to express more clearly what it was intended that the beneficiaries of care would receive from competent performance in the sector. However, the postal consultation provided feedback suggesting use of the term 'optimise', which was then reinstated into the key purpose, to give the phrase:

'To optimise their health and social well-being.'

Given the initial confusion of the term within the sector, we believe that this is a term which may still cause confusion to some and may need to be constantly reinterpreted for the particular setting in which the map is used.

The nature of the 'caring relationship'

Undoubtedly one of the greatest areas of debate in relation to the key purpose statement, and for the functional map as a whole, was the scope and nature of the main functions in the care sector and their definition.

In practice, three broad functions were defined:

- *Empowering* users so that both the initiative and the control of resources are in their control;
- *Enabling* users to deal with their health and social well-being needs – these functions depend on the practitioner/organisation taking the initiative (albeit in agreement/negotiation with the user) to make it possible for users to influence or alter what is on offer;

• *Intervening* (usually characterised by the words 'treat', 'protect', 'nurse' and so on) in order to deal directly with health and social well-being needs of users.

Some of the debate has been led by a concern that the map should not 'invent' or impose expectations on occupational groups which are inappropriate, which represent models now superseded in practice or which are desirable but unachievable in the current climate. Some of the concern appeared to stem from an unwillingness to recognise the breadth of the sector in its entirety with individuals not wishing, or not able, to acknowledge the work roles of others. In others, there was a concern that the terms used did not support the values and commitments which the sector promotes, albeit sometimes ineffectively.

When developing a functional map, one must make choices and these choices must be informed by whatever information on best practice can be gained. However, a map, above all else, must describe the sector as a whole. It is not the purpose of a map to propose solutions to disagreements or to ignore tensions that exist in the sector over what is expected of people. So, whilst the main issues were noted, the view was taken that the map should describe functions in terms of everyone's expectations, not just in terms of one group, organisation, association or generation. The authenticity of the map rests ultimately on whether it describes expectations that actually are, and will continue to be, placed on work roles, no matter how acceptable these may be to certain individuals or organisations.

Conceptualising 'care' was a considerable challenge. Differing views and perspectives result in differing definitions of what care is, including an insistence in some quarters that the word care is inappropriate since it carries connotations of 'doing to' rather than 'working with' people, and is consequently a deprivation of people's rights and can lead to manipulation. On the other hand, there are some groups for whom the word and the concept of care is central to their identity (such as the nursing profession). A functional map that did not use the term might disenfranchise those workers whose chief role is to 'care or tend to' those who are unable (either temporarily or permanently) to look after themselves. It would also seem a little strange if the *Care* Sector Consortium's map omitted reference to the term!

Using a word and having a working concept are, however, two different things. For the sector as a whole, 'care' has assumed a very wide meaning, embracing all those functions which are to do with enabling, empowering, intervening, supporting and comforting. To adopt such a wide definition is, of course, risky. It means that 'care in the community' might represent a different set of component functions compared with, say, 'acute hospital care'. This may seem to be a statement of the obvious. It serves here to remind us that the map, although it describes functions in care, assumes no standard definition of the term but sees it as a construct, the content of which may change according to context. In other words, if someone wishes to know what care means in terms of occupational competence, they need to look for a role and a context and then see what specific functions, identifiable within the map, are expected.

As the functions within the map are so broad and represent a wide range of functions which are carried out within the sector, the focus of the broad level descriptions is on 'optimising health and social well-being' which appears to be recognised by all. At further levels of detail of the map, the word 'care' has been used in two different ways:

1. To describe those functions which specifically relate to those areas of work where individuals are 'cared for' as they are unable, either temporarily or permanently, to care for themselves – here the word care has a very specific meaning;
2. In a global way, to describe all of the services and facilities which come under the auspices of the sector and therefore have as their purpose 'to optimise the health and social well-being of individuals, families, groups and communities'. In this latter sense, the use of the word care is the same as that in the title of the 'Care Sector Consortium' – a descriptor for the sector as a whole.

This is not to suggest that the prime purpose of the care sector is solely to 'care for individuals' but to recognise that the term 'care sector' is known and generally understood. The sector itself needs to know that within the global definition a wide variety of functions actually exist, spanning a spectrum of work.

For the key purpose statement, it seemed that the one function which applies across the sector as a whole is that of 'enabling'. This is partly because it can be seen as the middle ground between 'empowering' and 'intervening' but also it is due to a recognition that it applies to whatever is happening within the sector, such as by:

171

- Enabling through offering choice;
- Enabling through making choices on others' behalf;
- Enabling through developing in others the ability to make choices;
- Enabling through providing access to the resources and authority needed to make choices;
- and so on.

There also seemed to be the widely-held belief that practice is developing through enabling service users to make their own decisions about their health and social well-being and to take greater responsibility for it. This too reflects moves away from treatment towards the promotion of health and social well-being and a correspondingly greater focus on prevention and protection. However, some in the sector expressed concern that this was not only a good practice model of 'care' but stemmed as well from a desire to reduce resources. This focus on offering choice, together with the beneficiaries of the sector and the purpose for which the work is being undertaken, resulted in the first part of the key purpose:

'Enable individuals, families, groups and communities to optimise their health and social well-being.'

Conditions of actions within the sector

Throughout the development of the key purpose, respondents referred to the need within the sector to weigh up and make choices between a number of factors. For some, this area was relatively straightforward as they believed their actions were driven by 'what is best for the individual concerned'. For others, this was the driving force but there was an additional and over-riding concern in relation to resource constraints. That is, the objective was 'to optimise health and social well-being' but this could only be achieved within available resources. For still other groups, it was not a matter of only what is right for the individual, but for their family, the community in which they live and so on. Here the complexity of the sector is revealed particularly when groups of workers are charged with making choices as to when the needs of 'the community' or 'of society' must prevail over those of individuals. In short, this is a recognition that the needs and actions of individuals are not the only factor which must be taken into account but that these are set in the context of the needs and rights of others. This is the rationale underlying the inclusion of the conditional phrase:

'balancing their respective needs with those of wider society'.

The issue of resources was debated at length within the project and in one sense it can be seen as a non-issue. It is possible to enable individuals *only* through the use of available resources. (It is difficult to imagine how one does it through unavailable resources!) But there are at least three sub-texts which inform the debate:

- Arguments about who is responsible for using resources prudently;
- Controversy about the adequacy of available resources and the justice with which they are allocated;
- Concern about the distribution of power and its use to influence both the size and allocation of resources.

A functional map cannot settle these debates, but cannot ignore them either. So although, logically, it is a tautology to refer to resources, its inclusion serves to remind future standards developers that:

- there are issues of judgment and choice in this area which they will have to address;
- while many in the sector have the ideal of resources being unlimited, in reality they are not.

The outcome of this development work means that the key purpose statement can be applied to all individuals, groups and organisations within the sector (see Figure 8.2).

Values within the sector

The nature of the functional map as a description of work expectations means that it will embody value judgments. Over and above this, all work, however lofty or humble, brings with it moral choices – what is good, what is bad, what is a just decision, what is a fair assessment, what is the proper way to deal with others, and so on.

173

```
┌─────────────────────────────────────────────────────────────────┐
│                                                                   │
│  The purpose of the care sector        ⎫                          │
│                                        ⎪                          │
│  The purpose of each organisation      ⎪   Enable individuals, families, │
│  or agency in health and social care   ⎪   groups and communities to   │
│                                        ⎪   optimise their health and    │
│  The purpose of each department or     ⎬   social well being, balancing │
│  section within organisations          ⎪   their respective needs with  │
│                                        ⎪   those of wider society and the│
│  The purpose of health and social      ⎪   available resources          │
│  care workers                          ⎪                          │
│                                        ⎪                          │
│  The purpose of each individual        ⎭                          │
│  worker in health and social care                                 │
│                                                                   │
└─────────────────────────────────────────────────────────────────┘
```

Figure 8.2   The key purpose statement for all levels of work

Care in all its functions is concerned directly and indirectly with facing (not necessarily resolving) dilemmas in meeting users' needs. This raises questions as to who is best placed to define 'needs' to the planning dilemmas that arise when allocating resources to services. These choices arise as dilemmas, not because of the way in which services are organised, nor because of the extent of the resources available to meet needs, but because 'care' (however it is defined) seems to be realisable only through choosing which of several interests will be served – those of the individual or of the community at large; those of this individual or that; those of the client or the practitioner; those of people in a particular category, or those of the 'system'; those interests that satisfy the demands of policy, or those which meet the needs of specific immediate circumstances. It follows that no description of competence in the care sector could be complete without accounting for making choices – a function that is central to all activity.

When the Care Standards and Awards were developed, it was decided that the values which underpin and guide the work of the sector should be explicitly detailed in a unit with specific value-based outcomes – the Value Base Unit. In addition, outcomes related to the expression of values were specified in each of the functional units so that good practice is firmly embedded through-out the model.

This expression of values as being central to work expectations within the sector was taken as the starting point for the functional mapping project, although due to the high level of generality of the functional map the criteria of effective performance were not detailed. This found resonance with participants who wished to ensure that values were central to the map and vital to good practice. Earlier versions of the map captured 'values' through identifying it as a separate domain alongside other functions in the map. However, feedback from the postal consultation confirmed that setting a values function alongside other functions could be misleading. It could appear that this was only one of many functions, rather than over-arching the map, and its relationship to other functions would be lost. In the final map, the 'values function' has therefore been shown as essentially different from all the other functions – that is, as the filter through which all the other functions are put into practice.

Whose reality?

Throughout the development of the map there was debate about its 'political nature', which included the following range of issues:

- The perspective the map should adopt – should it reflect current government policy and programmes or an ideal view of what health and social care ought to be like?
- Acceptable and unacceptable constructs for describing the outcomes of care – at issue here is the power a map might have in reinforcing outmoded approaches to care if such functions are captured within it;
- The relative weight which should be attached to different functions, such as those which describe direct relationships with users, and those which are indirect.

During discussions at the consultative workshops and within the Consortium, it was agreed that the map had to reflect 'political reality' in the sense that the sector works within a legislative, economic and social framework which has a direct impact on the lives of users and care workers alike. So, for example, the map must acknowledge that there is a purchaser–provider split within the care sector which brings with it new roles. At the same time, it is possible within the map to specify those work roles which may be seen to challenge the current framework and the status quo and which have the overall aim of improving the health and social well-being of individuals, families, groups and communities. These decisions led to the development of the functional map in its final form. The key purpose is split into six domains as illustrated below.

At the heart of the sector are service users: the individuals, families, groups and communities for whom all care services are provided. Therefore at the core of the functional map is the Value Domain – the promotion of values of good practice which relate to working with and for these service users (Figure 8.3). These values are central to the work of the sector and underpin and promote good practice.

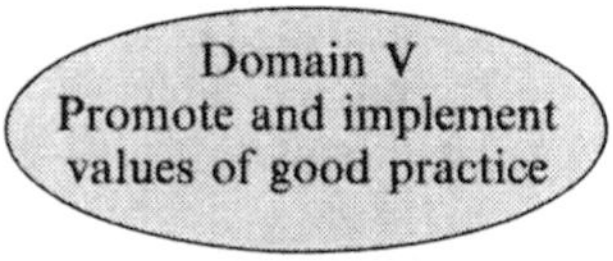

Domain V
Promote and implement
values of good practice

Figure 8.3   The value domain

Domains A and B (Figure 8.4) are the 'provider' roles and relate most closely to service users. It is these functions which distinguish the care sector from others as they describe direct interaction with individuals, families, groups and communities to optimise their health and social well-being. Domain A relates to those functions where individuals, families, groups and communities are enabled to take greater control over their health and social well-being by acquiring the necessary knowledge, skills and resources, influencing the environment in which they live and through minimising any risks. Domain B relates to those functions where there is a more direct intervention between the provider of services and the service user.

Individuals and organisations whose key purpose is to 'optimise the health and social well-being of individuals, families, groups and communities' need to be supported to improve their practice continually. This should be an interactive process, with innovations and improvements in practice stemming from one part of the sector, or one organisation, being communicated to others for the benefit of all. Domain C (Figure 8.5) describes the functions of improving

176

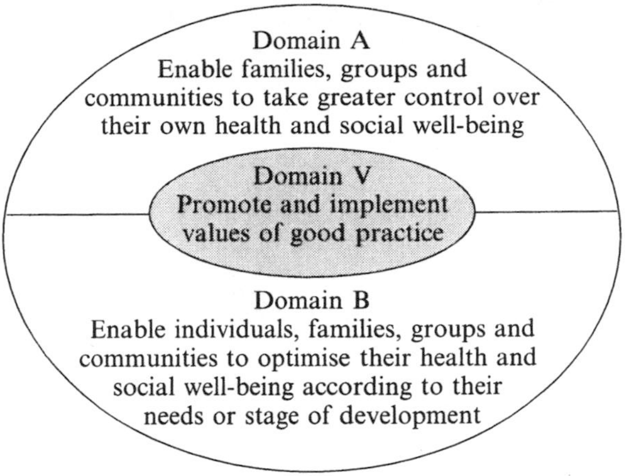

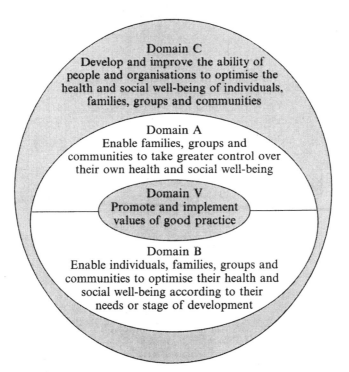

Figure 8.4   Adding the provider roles of domains A and B

Figure 8.5   Adding the knowledge and practice functions of domain C

177

knowledge and practice for the sector as a whole and has been positioned at the interface between the provider and commissioning functions, as it relates to both.

Domain D (Figure 8.6) describes commissioning, coordination and facilitation functions – those which can usually be thought of as 'organisational'. In the care sector, these functions may take place on a single or multi-agency basis. The commissioning functions are those which determine the services and facilities which are needed in

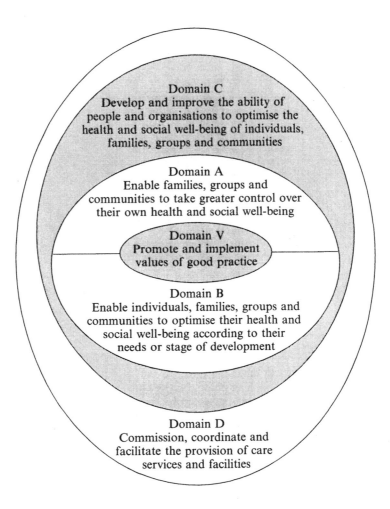

Figure 8.6   With the organisational function of domain D

a geographical area and the optimal allocation of resources to meet the health and social well-being needs of the population. Also within this domain, there is the coordination and development of provider services, and two key roles which are related to both the commissioning and providing roles – securing, developing and deploying resources, and supporting, facilitating and effecting the movement of people, information and resources.

The commissioning and provision of care services takes place within a strategic framework, shaped by an overall assessment of a population's needs and the development of targets, strategies and structures to meet those needs. This function is described by Domain E.

All functions of the sector take place within the national and international legislative, social, political, economic and environmental context, and are shown together in Figure 8.7.

The details of the analysis are available within the functional map document itself. (Copies of the functional map can be obtained direct from the Care Sector Consortium, 3 Devonshire Street, LONDON W1N 2BA. Tel: 0171 436 8712.)

Table 8.2 shows the first level of breakdown of the map from the domains A to E – the key roles. Within the map, each of the key roles is then broken down into one further level of analysis, the descriptions of which are at sufficient levels of detail to provide reference points for the units of competence, which form the basis of NVQs and SVQs.

POTENTIAL USES OF THE FUNCTIONAL MAP

Whilst the development of the map was interesting in its own right, it was developed for one particular purpose – as a planning tool for the CSC to coordinate and integrate the development of national occupational standards and from them, the structure and content of National (Scottish) Vocational Qualifications in the sector. The way of doing this is to recognise commonality of function and expectations where they occur, but also to recognise the particular contributions which different health and social care practitioners make.

However, there are many other purposes for which the map can be used and we have identified some of these below, although no doubt there may be more.

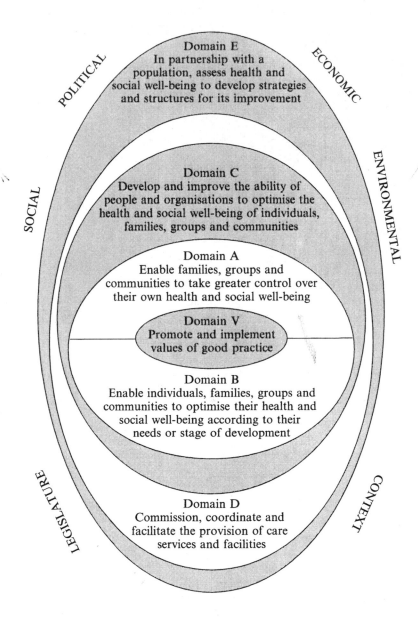

POLITICAL

ECONOMIC

SOCIAL

ENVIRONMENTAL

LEGISLATURE

CONTEXT

Domain E
In partnership with a population, assess health and social well-being to develop strategies and structures for its improvement

Domain C
Develop and improve the ability of people and organisations to optimise the health and social well-being of individuals, families, groups and communities

Domain A
Enable families, groups and communities to take greater control over their own health and social well-being

Domain V
Promote and implement values of good practice

Domain B
Enable individuals, families, groups and communities to optimise their health and social well-being according to their needs or stage of development

Domain D
Commission, coordinate and facilitate the provision of care services and facilities

Figure 8.7 All domains of the functional model

180

Table 8.2   The functional map: key purpose and first two tiers of analysis

Key purpose	Enable individuals, families, groups and communities to optimise their health and social well-being, balancing their respective needs with those of wider society and the available resources

V   Promote and
     implement values of
     good practice

		A1	Enable individuals, families, groups and communities to acquire the necessary knowledge, skills, confidence and resources to take greater control over their health and social well-being
A	Enable individuals, families, groups and communities to take greater control over their own health and social well-being	A2	Enable individuals, families, groups and communities to take greater control over their health and social well-being by influencing the environment in which they live
		A3	Enable individuals, families, groups and communities to take greater control over their health and social well-being by minimising the risk to themselves and others
		A4	Minimise and counteract the risk and harm caused to the health and social well-being of individuals, families, groups and communities by their own or others' behaviour
		B1	Assess with individuals, families, groups and communities their needs and options for optimising their health and social well-being and agree plans for how to do this
B	Enable individuals, families, groups and communities to optimise their health and social well-being according to their needs or stage of development	B2	Empower individuals, families, groups and communities to change, adjust to or come to terms with conditions within themselves, their social roles and develop their relationships with others
		B3	Enable individuals to develop their full potential and optimise their situation according to their needs or stage of development

181

Table 8.2 (*cont.*)

		B4	Enable individuals, families and groups to optimise their psychological and emotional functioning
		B5	Enable individuals to optimise their physical and sensory functioning and appearance
		B6	In agreement with individuals, seek to alleviate dysfunction, disease and symptoms in their physical and sensory functioning and appearance through the application of specific therapies
C	Develop and improve the ability of people and organisations to optimise the health and social well-being of individuals, families, groups and communities	C1	Extend knowledge and improve practice in optimising the health and social well-being of individuals, families, groups and communities
		C2	Develop, monitor and improve the practice of individuals whose purpose is to optimise the health and social well-being of individuals, families, groups and communities
		D1	Commission, evaluate and improve care services and facilities
D	Commission, coordinate and facilitate the provision of care services and facilities	D2	Coordinate and develop the provision of care services and facilities
		D3	Secure, deploy and develop resources to provide care services and facilities
		D4	Support, facilitate and effect the movement of people, information and products to, within and between care services and facilities
E	In partnership with a population, assess health and social well-being to develop strategies and structures for its improvement	E1	Investigate, monitor and evaluate the status and determinants of, and changes in, the health and social well-being of a population
		E2	Develop targets, strategies and structures for improving health and social well-being in partnership with a population

• The map can be used as a starting point for thinking about interprofessional working. By its nature, the map allows one to investigate where work roles and expectations are common and where they are similar but different. In essence, the functional map, and the national occupational standards developed from it, provide a common language through which issues of interprofessional working can be explored. At the time of writing this chapter, the CSC was in the process of commissioning three projects to develop occupational standards for professionals working in health care, all based on and planned from the functional map. These projects are in the areas of:

- the standards in common for six of the Professions Allied to Medicine in Post-Registration Practice – dietitians, occupational therapists, physiotherapists, podiatrists, radiographers, and speech and language therapists.
- Health Promotion – those for whom this is their specialist area of work and all those health and social care practitioners for whom this is only one part of their job;
- Complementary Medicine – the exemplar areas of aromatherapy, homeopathy, hypnotherapy and reflexology.

Each of these projects will not only be looking at the work roles that are common within each of these three project strands, but will also be seeking and recognising commonality across the whole programme of work. While this is a CSC project for the development of standards, it will contribute to interprofessional working as practitioners from the different professions join together to debate their work and recognise their common aims. The standards once developed will be capable of use in single and multi-disciplinary teams.

- The map can be used to inform the development of interprofessional qualifications providing public recognition for common areas of competence. Another CSC project is using the functional map as a coordination tool for reviewing all of the care sector NVQs/SVQs to make sure that they are contained within a common framework. Once all of the awards have been reviewed the aim is for a suite of care sector qualifications which will enable individuals to progress from one area of competence to another, as commonality of function is recognised. Common elements within currently different qualifications will be brought together into the one framework enabling the development of qualifications which are designed around the needs of groups of users, as well as those which reflect more traditional professional routes for development.
- The map may be of use in one's own personal and professional development – some of those engaged in the consultation on the

map found it to be 'energising', offering a fresh perspective on their work. This allowed them to reflect on the purpose and achievements of the service which they currently offered to users and provided a means of standing back and thinking through with others current aims and organisation. You could try this for yourself by using the functional map as a tool for thinking though what the sector is about. Does the map ring true for you? What parts of the map group together to form your current job? Could the roles in the map be better organised in your locality to offer an improved service to clients?

When the map has been developed into more levels of greater detail, and particularly when national occupational standards are available, then these can be used as a focus for discussion with those who work in the same sort of job as you, or with those who work in different but connecting jobs, to discuss whether you agree on the work expectations described and whether they characterise the service you are offering to users.

- The map having been used as a strategic planning tool by the CSC to develop national occupational standards, may then be of use in purchasing services for users and in contracting for those services. For example, purchasers may ask: What do we want our services to deliver to meet the needs of the service users in this area? How will we achieve a shift away from illness to focus on health and what does this mean for the work roles for those in the services we purchase? How might we use these descriptions within our contracts to ensure that we are purchasing the services we actually want?

WHAT NEXT?

The functional map focuses on the values and key concepts which underpin health and social care and describes the work roles which are necessary for delivering an effective service to meet the needs of all service users. It has a particular role to play in the design of occupational standards, and from them, the development of quali-fications. The CSC, the lead body charged with taking the work forward in these areas for the care sector as a whole, is already using the map extensively for these purposes.

But we might question whether the map can, or should, be used for other purposes as well. Could it, and should it, be used, for example, to:

- influence national policies on health and social care?
- improve the quality of care for service users by focusing on their needs and by providing them with the range of services they might expect to receive?
- improve interprofessional working and development?

These questions are as important for you to answer as they are for us, and so we leave it for you to think about and debate . . .

CHAPTER NINE

Interprofessional Collaboration: Problems and Prospects

Simon Biggs

WHAT IS INTERPROFESSIONAL COLLABORATION: EXPLORING THE HINTERLAND

Interprofessional collaboration is often spoken of as 'a good thing' by policy makers, without examining possible differences of interpretation in greater detail. In reality, it can refer to a variety of practices and relationships that form a sort of hinterland of meaning behind policy objectives. If these differences are not clarified, misunderstandings can multiply. Implicit assumptions held by participants then come into sharp relief as policy statements have to be translated into operations.

This chapter will outline some of these interpretations, then examine recent social policy initiatives on interprofessionalism, its direction and some of its implications.

Taking 'Interprofessional' first, the term may be used to imply relationships other than those strictly obtaining between professional groups. For example, it may refer to relations between agencies (interagency) or within teams that have members from different disciplines within them (multidisciplinary). It is worth spending a little time examining these related, but distinctive, forms of collaboration before moving on.

Interprofessional, then, refers to relations between different professional groups. These might include medicine, nursing, professions allied to medicine, social work, police, probation, management and administration amongst others. Each one will have a distinctive professional culture which depends, by degrees, on established professional bodies and training and accrediting organisations. Handy (1985) has pointed out that it is a characteristic of staff in mature organisations that they have professional allegiances which cross-cut institutional boundaries. In other words, professional associations serve as anchors, reflecting and informing professional identity beyond identification with any one workplace. Professional identity may also be maintained by contrasting the characteristics of one's own group with other, or 'out-groups' (Turner, 1991). So, relations within any one workplace, or objectives that span workplaces, will need to take account of the fact that there will be different professional groups working within the same organisation/agency, and the same professional groups existing across different organisations/agencies.

Interagency collaboration refers to relations between different organisations/agencies. These may or may not consist of staff drawn primarily from a single professional group. For example, whilst social service departments recruit heavily in favour of social work, NHS bodies employ staff from a variety of professional backgrounds. Different agencies might also belong to different sectors, such as the NHS, local authorities, voluntary and private care. Separate agencies tend to develop their own cultures, manifested in their policies and procedures, which contribute to a sense of their primary task (what they are there to do). Agencies may also have different, and on occasion competing, funding arrangements.

Multidisciplinary working refers to teams or more fluid working arrangements (networks, interest groups). These entities consist of members from different professional groups, but who are working towards a specific and sharply focused goal. For example, Ingrid Barker's study of social work roles in such teams states, 'What we are concerned with here is the social worker's place in a team made up of different professionals, sharing common objectives and based (at least some of the time) in the same building' (Barker, 1989, p. 8).

The context, then, is focused, enduring and tends to be small-scale, either a small agency or a unit within a larger agency. Such contexts would allow expression of distinctive professional contributions, whilst contributing to shared identity.

If the first semantic hurdle consists of the meaning implied by interprofessional, a second, the meaning of collaboration, is subject to similar fuzziness. Hallett and Birchall (1992) have noted that different terms have commonsense meanings that are closely related. They identify collaboration, coordination and cooperation as forms of combination that are often confused. This confusion is reflected in social policy. For example, Weiss (1981) notes that coordination is:

'discussed in the political arena as though everyone knows precisely what it means, when in fact it means many inconsistent things and occasionally means nothing at all'.
(p. 41)

Cooperation implies 'working together' with positive connotations, but was not pursued in Hallett and Birchall's review of terminology.

Coordination connotes that separate groups take the activities of other groups into account (Hall *et al.*, 1977) in order to ensure compatibility and deal collectively with a shared task. Collaboration (Dartington, 1986) describes working together to achieve something which neither agency could achieve alone.

Each implies different degrees of closeness and protectiveness of the professional or agency base.

Whilst each interpretation of interprofessionalism gives it a different slant, it is possible to identify similar tensions and concerns across them. These similarities are centred around the question of identity and, most notably, between loss of identity through immersion in a wider and less well-defined group, or by being swamped by a more dominant group.

The security of identity will influence how far merger with a larger group, be that joining an interprofessional environment or working for a particular agency, is perceived as threatening. It will also be affected by an opposite concern, how far separateness leads to professional isolation and an inability to collaborate around shared tasks and objectives. Tasks associated with successful negotiation of this conflict will vary depending on some of the definitions noted earlier. Interprofessional collaboration might centre on how far the unique contributions of each discipline are enhanced and rivalry reduced.

Interagency collaboration may depend upon how far a coherent service can be provided to users in a shared location, or target group, which does not eclipse the guiding principles of each participating organisation. Multidisciplinary collaboration may require that centripuntal forces, those drawing professionals with different backgrounds into a team, are balanced against centrifugal ones, pulling them towards a purist and separate professional identity.

Each addresses the question of identity and loyalty: to a particular professional ethos, to an agency's mission, or to end-users of a service. These identities need not necessarily be in competition; in the best contexts, they should enable practitioners to work in harmony. What, then, does this semantic hinterland tell us about interprofessionalism? Largely that the concept is imprecise. It may thus become prey to the influence of different policy and practice environments.

In summary, success will depend upon the correct balance being achieved between the maintenance of separate identities, merging to fulfil a shared objective and the resolution of possibly conflicting loyalties. Interprofessional collaboration will depend on the recognition of difference, interdependence and shared objectives.

In the next section I will examine how different social policy environments have fashioned our understanding of interprofessionalism, its form and the value attributed to it.

SOCIAL POLICY INITIATIVES ON INTERPROFESSIONALISM

The need for closer attention to interprofessional relations has been felt in both children's and adults' services. In children's services, a number of inquiries had, by the late 1980s, identified a lack of coordination across both professions and agencies. A failure to protect children was associated with missed information, abetted by gaps in communication between professional groups in different organisations.

Around the same time, there was growing awareness that adults' services were often confusing to the client/patient/end-user, particularly in community settings. If lots of different services are coming in, from different agencies, interventions need to be 'coherent, consistent and well planned' (Department of Health, 1991). Further, personally tailored care packages were to be recommended as a consequence of assessment of individual need, rather than assessment for a particular service. These packages of care would require coordination between professionals offering parts of the overall service.

Finally, it needs to be said that concern about the coordination of services is not new to British social policy. The Beveridge Report (1942), for example, included explicit acknowledgement of the interdependence of policies for full employment, social security and comprehensive health care. Such macro-level coordination was recognised in the Seebohm Report's (1968) recommendation that services for children, mental health and welfare of adults should be unified under the auspices of local authorities. Whilst the separation between health and social care remained, attempts were made in succeeding years to coordinate activities. Joint planning was included within the NHS Reorganisation Act of 1973 with joint finance following shortly in 1976. The expansion of private care following the 1979 election and the distinction between purchasers and providers arising from the 1990 NHS and Community Care Act both added to the dimensions of interagency collaboration required, and gave impetus to further joint approaches, particularly between purchasing authorities.

THE CHILDREN ACT 1989

Whilst interprofessional collaboration is not writ large in the Act itself (for example it is not mentioned amongst the 42 principles of good child care practice in 'The Care of Children' (1989), Department of Health guidance to the Act), it has featured strongly in both the lead up to 1989 and in subsequent policy concerns. The Jasmine Beckford Inquiry (Blom-Cooper, 1985) emphasised the importance of communication between agencies and professional groups, most notably social work and community health services. Following the Cleveland Inquiry (Butler-Sloss, 1988), more complex and more precise issues began to emerge as 'an honest attempt was made to address problems between agencies' prior to the scandal taking place. It occasioned the publication of guidance by the Department of Health (Home Office, D of H, DES, Welsh Office (1991) Working Together Under the Children Act 1989, HMSO London) to coincide with the Inquiry report itself. This guidance was revised in 1991 by the Home Office and includes the statement: 'Inter-disciplinary and inter-agency work is an essential process in the professional task of attempting to protect children from abuse' (p. 53). The source of this revised publication was not accidental, and reflects a trend towards increased legalism in child protective practice (see Otway and Parton, 1995). Interprofessional collaboration in child care is, then, as much about criminal justice systems as the more 'traditional' concern with health and welfare. As a result, an increased reliance on procedural detail and coordination, plus

the need to obtain evidence uncontaminated by professio.
pretation or the influencing of vulnerable witnesses, has
managerial approach to much of this work.

Whatever the balance of forces between different interests i
care and protection, the underlying policy thrust has ass..ned
distinctive contributions from discrete professional groups who
use their complementary skills to approach an agreed task. Whilst
subject to boundary dispute and leadership questions, the overall
feel is one of stability with relatively little threat to the core
identities of the professional groups or agencies involved.

THE NHS AND COMMUNITY CARE ACT 1990

Whilst the Children Act has been interpreted as requiring closer
collaboration between distinct and complementary professional
groups and agencies, the 1990 NHS and Community Care Act
(Department of Health, 1990) can be seen to stretch our subject in
different directions. The encouragement of a mixed welfare economy has led to increased diversity of services, most notably between
statutory, voluntary and private sectors. This has been counter-
balanced by trends towards generalism in terms of management,
quality systems and an enhanced awareness of commonality between the skills required from different professional groups. In
terms of policy, once the induction of competition had succeeded in
fragmenting community services between sectors, some way had to
be found to put Humpty together again. An underlying principle of
the 1990 act includes: 'services which are integrated in such a way
that users experience them as coherent, consistent and well planned,
despite the fact that a number of agencies will be involved'
(Department of Health, 1991, p. 1).

The practical implications of this and other requirements manifested themselves in two additional ways. First, a strategic concern
with 'jointness' and in particular the integration of health and
welfare planning and service delivery. This objective has been
fortified by funding being made contingent on the achievement of
shared purchasing strategies. Second, attempts were made to promote a generic community care worker. This second policy desire
had its roots at the beginnings of the community care reforms. The
Griffiths Report (1988) suggested the adoption of 'case management' as a role that could be undertaken by staff from a variety of
professional backgrounds, and echoed Audit Commission recom-

mendations that 'a new occupation of "community carers"... be created ... to undertake the front line personal and social support of dependent people' (Griffiths, 1988; paragraph 8.4).

These three wishes, for coherence at the point of delivery, coordination at the point of purchasing and genericism at the point of professional intervention, can be seen as coming together in the policy demand, most vocal in the early 1990s, for a 'seamless service'. The means of addressing the problem of interprofessional collaboration showed tendencies to abolish it by promoting an increasingly generic approach.

In comparison to children's services, community care reforms in the 1990s have placed greater strain on the balance between professional and agency-based identity. This process has had both unifying and diversifying effects on interprofessionalism, which will be explored shortly.

WHY INTERPROFESSIONALISM?

It is a curious point that whilst all of the policy documents mentioned above clearly approve of closer interprofessional collaboration, this is often presented as a self-evident truth and little is done by way of persuasive argument to convince the reader of the pros and cons of such a policy goal or, indeed, whether it can deliver the outcomes that have become associated with it.

Hallett and Birchall (1992) have summarised the policy goals that have been associated with greater coordination which they refer to as the 'optimistic tradition' in this field. These are said to include the following:

- The achievement of greater efficiency in the use of resources, and improved standards of service delivery through the avoidance of duplication and overlap in service provision;
- Reduction of gaps and discontinuities in services;
- The clarification of roles and responsibilities, arising in 'frontier problems' and demarcation disputes between professions and services;
- The delivery of comprehensive, holistic services.
  (p.17)

The promotion of a service driven by objectives and outcomes rather than by professional interests could be added to this list, as could an attempt to replace relatively well-paid professional staff with more closely supervised, but less expensive ancillaries.

However, a number of writers have questioned whether inter-professional collaboration can achieve these objectives and point to factors that might conflict with other policy objectives.

It could, for example, be argued that closer links between professions and between agencies can reduce choice for users of services. This would happen, for example, if the opportunities for alternative assessments for users' requirements were reduced. Standardised forms of assessment, or single point of entry assessment to a multidisciplinary system, would mean that wherever you went as a user of services you would get the same answer. Diversity is lost, not simply in terms of assessment but also in terms of the services themselves if each is delivered through the same multidisciplinary network.

The integrity of interprofessionalism has also been questioned in terms of the effects of shared information on individual liberties (Dingwall, 1983; Domoney et al., 1989). Whilst confidentiality within professions or agencies has often been portrayed as a stumbling block to collaboration, sharing of information could lead to the labelling of individuals requiring services and to collusion between professionals against the client. Interprofessionalism would, according to this argument, act as an accelerator for negative attributions within service systems, which would be very difficult to challenge from the outside.

Further, collective definitions of problems and their solutions might militate against 'risky' or novel solutions. Conservatising tendencies within professional judgement would limit choice to existing services (Parton, 1985).

Finally, a focus on interprofessionalism, particularly in terms of service planning, is inward-looking in so far as attention is being paid to the different parts of a service system and its integration as a system (Biggs, 1990). This might eclipse consideration of macro-system problems external to the agencies concerned. An example of such a focus would be to attribute the failure to solve social problems to the need for ever greater collaboration between services rather than extrinsic factors such as poverty, poor housing, a punitive moral climate and so on. An undue emphasis on collaboration under these conditions might thereby fail to address whether professional effort was going into the right areas to address the problem, and whether the resources available were significant enough to have an impact.

193

An overview of policy and practice issues around interprofessionalism has indicated that current contexts include tendencies that are at one and the same time unifying and leading to diversity. The former is perhaps most evident within agencies, with considerable emphasis on the latter in the distribution of services. These trends are most evident in community care for adults, and, by dint of reorganisations, seepage from one service to another and changing funding arrangements, they have a significant influence for other service user groups.

UNIFYING TENDENCIES: GENERAL MANAGEMENT AND QUALITY CONTROL

Unifying tendencies within service systems may place strain on professional identity and it is worth considering them in greater detail.

When Griffiths reviewed adult services in 1988, he was quoted as saying:

'If Florence Nightingale were carrying her lamp through the corridors of the NHS today, she would almost certainly be searching for the people in charge.'
(Times, 30 March 1994)

Thus one of the key changes to contemporary health and welfare was bound to be the development of general management in line with practice in commercial sectors.

General management is intended to operate across all disciplines and functions. It can be seen as an attempt to get away from the 'tribalism of health service trades'. As such, this change would inevitably lead to conflict concerning previous emphasis on 'clinical responsibility' held by the medical profession, and enshrined at the beginning of the NHS (Nurse, 1993). General management also places a unified identity at the centre of organisation development, particularly when it is identified with an 'excellence' approach to management through quality control (Pfeiffer and Coote, 1991). Senior management identify a mission, a vision, which all workers sign up to. According to this model, excellence relies heavily on leadership and all workers have a stake in the success of the enterprise. It is thus a top-down approach, with little room for

194

alternative allegiancies or power bases which may compete with the mission. This is because a successful mission is seen as being closely related to survival in an increasingly competitive environment.

A concomitant to this approach is the construction of clear structures, objectives and defined responsibilities. Outcomes of services, rather than the inputs of different professional groups, are seen as central to an assessment of service effectiveness. If a service can achieve the same, or better outcomes, using groups of workers who do not traditionally perform certain tasks, then this is seen as more important than the contribution of particular group interests. The criterion for effectiveness changes from 'who does what' to 'what gets done'.

A second demand, following from increasing competition, would be to increase flexibility by contracting services out. This makes it much easier for the management core of an organisation to change with changing external demands, both in terms of selecting different providers of services if quality is not sufficient at a given price, or if customer requirements change.

These unifying tendencies thus pull strongly towards merger with management tasks, whilst simultaneously threatening fragmentation of previous identities. There is thus a structural and economic change implied in the position of helping professionals. If they find themselves on the providing side of the purchaser/provider equation, they are subject to competitive contracting against fellow professionals, which would break down within-professional allegiances. On the other hand, objective or outcome-driven decision-making, rather than that based on sectional interests, would place identification with the agency mission at a premium for both purchasers and providers. Again, professional identification would be reduced.

Thus, the influence of general management and competition slants expectations towards merger and away from the fostering of independent professional identities. Considerable pressure would be placed on established professional identities and make the management of boundaries between professional groups, and between them and general management, problematic.

In summary, managerialism and quality issues have provoked a strong alternative unifying pole of attraction for identity, backed up by financial clout. Further, the move has been towards management, not administration. In other words it is about the control of, rather than servicing the work of, other professional groups. The vectors within the system simultaneously foster a fragmentation of existing professional groups and integration across traditional professional boundaries.

DIVERSIFYING TENDENCIES: USER PARTICIPATION AND INDIVIDUAL NEED

The 'seamless service' draws on the view that users are not so much concerned with issues of interdisciplinary demarcation, but in receiving a service that is both effective and efficient. By implication, services should be 'needs-led' with individualised requirements as the criterion for services rather than a 'fitting in' with existing arrangements.

At first glance, a movement towards 'seamlessness' might be thought to further increase pressure towards merger, and thus threaten professional identity. A more subtle analysis of the forces at play shows that participation also holds the seeds of re-establishing the primary goals of caring systems (Biggs, 1993b) and the part each profession can play within them. These might otherwise be lost in the momentum towards internal policy and procedure implied by general management. Such underlying trends would strengthen both professional expertise and interprofessionalism. The paradox of general management in health and welfare is that in order to establish quality outcome measures, considerable attention has to be paid to the mechanisms and coordinative activities within organisations. The danger is, then, that an emphasis on interprofessionalism might intensify intra-organisational negotiation at the cost of attention to the requirements of patients and other service users. In other words, boundary transactions within agencies come to take up energy and resources that would eclipse what is actually going on at the point of service delivery, the primary point of contact with the customers, consumers and end-users of the service (Biggs, 1990).

I have argued elsewhere (Biggs, 1993a) that user-involvement provides an antidote to such internalising trends for the following reasons:

1. A focus on user-participation re-establishes the point of delivery, where service users and staff interact, as the principle focus for decision-taking.

2. It makes the 'primary goal' of caring and healing much more visible in the day-to-day workings of an agency. It is less likely to get lost amongst the toing and froing of interprofessional or managerial negotiation inside and between agencies.

3. Both of the preceding points would significantly enhance the likelihood of the managerial mission and professional expertise developing in harness, rather than in competition. This is, in part, because most professionals find that their original motivation, loosely conceived as 'helping people', or 'working with people', is confirmed at the same time as managers can put meaningful substance into the rather abstract structures they have been trying to implement.

To these points can be added the view that a coordination of specialised professional inputs around individual requirements of service-users allows interprofessionalism to establish a 'superordinate goal' (Sherif, 1954). Superordinate goals provide an overarching reason for collaboration that is greater than the particular needs of any one participating group. It is thus easier to keep an agreed 'why' for collaboration in focus and not get lost in professional rivalry. That the focus has also shifted back to expertise that users require, can also bolster professional practice and thus significantly reduce the threatening elements of merger.

Increasing diversity may then be able to progress hand in hand with a measured sense of professional purpose. For this optimistic scenario to develop, it is crucial that users also come to be seen as expert. They are expert in the sense of holding unique knowledge of the consumption of services. It is, in other words, when one uses a service that attention is drawn to its gaps, discontinuities and general lack of fit with the requirements it is intended to fulfil.

TOWARDS SECURITY AND CHANGE

A question raised by this analysis is the degree to which interprofessional collaboration enhances the attainment of the primary goals of public services as they relate to their end-users or customers, and how far it can become a means of avoiding problems that are perceived to be insoluble. How far, then, is interprofessionalism allowed by its surrounding circumstances to become outward looking, and how far does it become inward looking?

For interprofessionalism to successfully achieve an improved service, policy makers must pay considered attention to the balance within professional identities. If pressures to merge are too great and identities too fragile, service development runs the risk of producing opposite reactions to those intended. Pressure to merge can as easily increase rivalry between groups for status and resources. It might foster alliances, but ones which run counter to the objectives of the whole agency. It may create a new 'in-group' (people like us) across helping professionals who can now see a common enemy, or 'out-group', in general management that is threatening to established identity structures. Success would depend on the following which, whilst not an exhaustive list, would both contribute to the maintenance of security and foster positive change:

- A recognition of specialist expertise as the necessary core of professional identity and purpose. This would ensure that each collaborator had a significant and valued contribution to make to the established task. It would form the ground upon which experiments in interprofessionalism can begin.
- A recognition that outcomes can be achieved only by a combination of different inputs; that, generally speaking, health and welfare tasks are simply too complex to be successful using the skills of a single profession.
- That, in the final analysis, each profession including management and administration is working towards a shared primary goal.
- To achieve meaning, the primary goal must be grounded by the participation of end-users in decision-taking at a variety of levels within agencies or collaborating agencies.

CONCLUSIONS

UK policy in the late 1980s and early 1990s has asked the question 'what is wrong with services?' rather than what problems need tackling in the outside world. In future it should re-focus on how partnerships between the users of services, professional workers and managers can be achieved. In other words 'how can we make an integrated service truly democratic?'

In organisational terms, if relatively stable and mature organisations promote the development of professions with independent values and identities, periods of upheaval, fragmentation, casualisation of labour through the contract culture, tend to diminish the power of such allegiances in favour of allegiance to competing agencies. Tendencies towards managerialism and, in particular, certain interpretations of quality management, enhance the rewards of changed allegiances but have also increased the risks of noncompliance. Future efforts towards interprofessional collaboration must build on the strengths of management coordination, professional expertise and increased user-participation. It will then become both efficient and effective and might even be able to deliver services that people need in ways that they want.

References

Barker, I. (1989) *Multidisciplinary Teamwork.* London: Central Council for Education and Training in Social Work.

Beveridge, W. (1942) *Social Insurance and Allied Services,* Cm. 6404. London: HMSO.

Biggs, S. (1990) Consumers, case management and inspection: obscuring social deprivation and need? *Critical Social Policy,* 30, pp. 23–38.

Biggs, S. (1993a) User participation and interprofessional collaboration in community care. *Journal of Interprofessional Care,* 7(2), pp. 151–9.

Biggs S. (1993b) *Understanding Ageing: Images Attitudes and Professional Practice.* Buckingham: Open University Press.

Blom-Cooper, L. (1985) *A Child in Trust:* The report of the panel of inquiry into the circumstances surrounding the death of Jasmine Beckford. London: Brent.

Butler-Sloss, L. (1988) *Report into the Inquiry into Child Abuse in Cleveland, 1987,* Cm. 412, London: HMSO.

Dartington, T. (1986) *The Limits to Altruism.* London: King's Fund.

Department of Health (1989a) *Caring for People: Community Care in the Next Decade and Beyond,* Cm. 849. London: HMSO.

Department of Health (1989b) *The Children Act: An Introductory Guide for the NHS.* London: HMSO.

Department of Health (1990) The NHS and Community Care Act. London: HMSO.

Department of Health (SSI) (1991) *Training for Community Care A Joint Approach.* London: HMSO.

Dingwall, R. (1983) Working together. *Maternal and Child Health*, April, pp. 153–7.

Domoney, L., Smale, G. and Warwick, J. (1989) *Shared Care*. London: National Institute of Social Work.

Griffiths, R. (1988) *Community Care: Agenda for Action*. London: HMSO.

Hall, R. (1977) *Organisations: Structure and Process*. New Jersey: Prentice Hall.

Hallett, C. and Birchall, E. (1992) *Coordination and Child Protection*. London: HMSO.

Handy, C. (1985) *Understanding Organisations*. London: Penguin.

Home Office, DoH, DES, Welsh Office (1991) *Working Together Under the Children Act 1989*. London: HMSO.

Nurse, J. (1993) The decline (and fall?) of professional influence in the NHS. *Journal of Interprofessional Care*, 7(2) pp. 131–40.

Otway, O. and Parton, N. (1995) *The contemporary state of child protection policy and practice in England and Wales*, New Directions in Social Work. London: Routledge.

Parton, N. (1985) *The Politics of Child Abuse*. London: Macmillan.

Pfeiffer, N. and Coote, A. (1991) *Is Quality Good for You?* London: Institute for Public Policy Research.

Seebohm Report (1968) Report of the Committee on Local Authority and Allied Personal Social Services, Cmnd. 3703, HMSO, London.

Sherif, M. (1954) *Experimental Study of Positive and Negative Intergroup Attitudes between Experimentally Produced Groups*. Norman, Oklahoma: Strong and Robinson.

Turner, J. C. (1991) *Social Influence*. Open University Press, Bucks.

Weinstein, J. (1994) *Sewing the Seams for a Seamless Service*, London: Central Council for Education and Training in Social Work.

Weiss, J. (1981) Substance v. symbol in administrative reform: the case for human services coordination. *Policy Analysis*, 7(1) pp. 21–45.

CHAPTER TEN

The World Health Organisation and European Union: Occupational, Vocational and Health Initiatives and their Implications for Cooperation Amongst the Professions

Tony Thompson and Peter Mathias

INTRODUCTION

There can be little doubt that the uncertainty which epitomises the world of work today as experienced by professionals is the direct result of the interaction of a wide variety of conflicting changes in economic conditions, social values, rapid information flows, technological changes and those associated with the socio-political scene. The origins of many of these changes lie in:

- demand for better choice and better quality of service provision;
- the demand for market share and jobs from evolving provider competition across geographic boundaries;
- demands for equality;
- demands for improved social and environmental conditions together with adequate rewards for the work undertaken.

In the last decade professionals have been under particular pressure to balance the risks and opportunities which can arise from the demands associated with change, but this balancing act is tricky as it involves an understanding of the many features of change which are interrelated and highly complex.

In this chapter:

1. general influences on the professions and their cooperation will be identified;
2. broad influences emerging from the European Community will be analysed;
3. European Vocational Policies will be described;
4. the work of the World Health Organisation will be introduced;
5. the *Health for All* targets and their implications will be reviewed.

The professions have experienced many of the effects associated with the removal of barriers to competition that trade and industry have felt; effects which may improve trade and labour opportunities but which at the same time can threaten employment and welfare protection, health and safety protection and other methods of safeguarding specific interests. The contemporary technologies which are assisting new products, new services and different methods of working have created risks and challenges which may have far-reaching social implications. As the pressures for change mount and the pace of competition within the services accelerates, then the professions and organisations which have held the monopoly on services may well find that they have to face tremendous demands to add value to their services in order for their members to survive. It may well be that the challenges which have resulted from conflicting demands, such as the increasing job insecurity in the more developed world, the high levels of stress induced problems and the uncertain future that even professionals find themselves having to face, could bring about a different type of expectation in relation to the way those professionals work in order to provide a service.

The previous cult of individualism could have spawned the growth in making professions assess the level and spread of their own resources and might lead us to consider that the professions cannot and maybe do not want to survive entirely alone any more than do individuals in society. The socio-political culture which is emerging within the United Kingdom during the late 1990s is possibly an indication that a more informed understanding of needs in relation to other groups is likely to emerge. There are numerous reasons why the professions have to become less inwardly focused, and more public about their limitations. But as this phenomenon emerges, it is likely that the sharing of experiences and values in order to get things right could result in better ways to provide services and to solve problems together as practitioners.

More effective levels of cooperation and collaboration, together with strategic working, will be required if the global problems associated with health and social care provision are to be tackled with optimism.

PUSHING AT THE RANGE OF PROFESSIONAL COMPETENCE

Reform of the health and social care system is high on most political agendas of the European countries. These reforms tend to include amongst others, structural and organisational changes in the delivery of the services, the introduction of market mechanisms into public sector agencies, and enhanced methods for containing costs and making services more user-focused. Quite often the changes are those which pushed developments in the health and social field towards primary care delivery and a reconfiguration of the acute care services. Such developments have brought in their wake a drive for more cost effective training solutions which have led to better provision of individualised and modular learning, computer based training, distance and open learning.

In some instances the methodologies have been found to be cheaper per unit cost, particularly when applied to the more time-consuming or repetitive training activities. Further, they are less likely to be disruptive to work schedules since they allow flexibility in terms of timing and access. The assessibility of digital transmission and storage of text, sound and graphics with moving pictures and the tremendous improvement in these systems now allow the development of multimedia training applications of great sophistication. In turn, education and training providers, both public and private, are incorporating these new training methodologies into their programmes thereby increasing the range of opportunities for self-development and the acquisition of transferable skills. It is the notion of transferable skills that may well be seen to be the factor that during the late 1990s has put the care professions into a state of transition. Professions within the care sectors are becoming increasingly like those in the commercial and industrial world, in that they are acquiring new skills to make the most of challenges and opportunities offered by ever greater demand and expectations of the purchasers.

The revolution in the services of the late 1980s and the on-going erosion of professional status has certainly come as quite a shock to many professionals. There is now an increasing realisation that the maintenance of technical proficiency is no longer enough, and members of the care professions are required to address the issues associated with the growing importance of developing a range of skills which include networking and marketing, negotiation, value added client care, project management, team and cross functional skills. The strategic policies which are emerging in health and social care within Europe are in turn demanding the translation of this awareness into competent action in the future.

During the next 10 years it is likely that there will be a major transition which will bring along different opportunities, strengths, weaknesses and threats to the professions. Some of the effects of the transition are already being felt and can be seen in the fact that in the developed world there are over 35 000 000 people who are unemployed. Of this total more than half of these are within the European landmass. There is a raging debate amongst strategists who now agree that it is important to balance market forces and social responsibility, and this is reflected in the arguments of the advocates of social responsibility and the controlled developments or otherwise of the interactions of the free market. In the United Kingdom the introduction of measures such as the European Community's social chapter is an indication of the elements of such arguments. The professional carers have to extend the depth and breadth of their existing knowledge and the range of their skills or face the prospects of seeing the results of failing to adapt and watching others exploit the reserves of skill transfer.

In order to cope with the fast change in the professional environment, workers are being required to develop new abilities which include those associated with living with doubt and uncertainty, whilst at the same time promoting a positive view to the service users. In the health and social care sector it is likely that the professionals will be continued to expect to work harder and longer and at the same time accept increasing accountability whilst working to higher standards. They will certainly be expected to update their skills on a more frequent basis than has hitherto been the case. Professions will have to respond to service demands by encompassing elements that extend beyond their immediate competence requirements of their current employment.

The key changes in the health and social care domains no longer fit neatly into traditional subject pigeon-holes; they tend to traverse the whole curriculum and hence require interdisciplinary approaches to education and training. They demand skills of the professionals which are not the narrow cognitive and subject-specific ones with which the professions have been traditionally equipped. In future the outcomes of courses will require professionals to consider aspects which are broader than procedural ones, for example the environmental and societal consequences of the profession's activities. In future, then, education and training associated with responding to health and care targets must offer the developing professional the skills to adapt to change and concentrate on the fundamental principles which are likely to underpin the development of specialist expertise. Naturally, this will mean that professions will have to be prepared to stray outside of their traditional boundaries. They will have to work as inter-disciplinary teams in planning and delivering the service. Integrative strategies of working will have to be developed and the teaching of these will have to go beyond mere cognitive skills, and assessment strategies will have to be developed which match all of these demands.

THE DEMANDING INTERNATIONAL DIMENSIONS FOR CARE PRACTICE

Many of the health and public policy initiatives which are affecting the way professionals work at the moment are rooted in the activities of the European Community. This Community is a unique grouping of member states which are committed to economic, social and political integration. They have a combined population of over 350 million, and they form the world's largest trading entity apart from being a growing force for democracy and peaceful international cooperation in the world at large.

The aims of the Community are set out in its founding treaties which are essentially economic. These revolve around activities which create a single economic region in which goods, services, people and capital can move as freely as they do within their own national boundaries. However, the creation of the European Community was also an act of political will. Its founders saw it as opening the way to 'an ever closer union among the people of Europe'. During the last decade of this century the Community is moving towards the full implementation of the single market as well as closer economic and political union. The history of its foundation is important as it was born in the aftermath of the Second World War. It was this war that resulted in millions of deaths and in the physical and economic destruction of a large part of Europe. A Community was established to ensure peace in Europe, to preserve democracy and to develop a firm economic base and political influence.

Through the various treaties which set up the Community, the member states which compose it have given Institutions the power to act, and to legislate at a European level in specified economic, social and other areas. The unique nature of the European Community is reflected in its four governing Institutions; the Council of Ministers, the European Parliament, the Commission and the Court of Justice. The Council of Ministers is the major decision-making body. The Council consists of one minister from each of the member states with the participating ministers varying according to the topic under discussion.

The European Commission, with headquarters in Brussels, is responsible for drafting proposals for community legislation. It is both the Community's Executive Body and its main Civil Service. The basic process of legislation is that the Council takes a decision on a Commission proposal after it has been scrutinised and amended in the European Parliament.

It was originally agreed by the member states that consideration of any enlargement of the European Community would have to wait until the single market was firmly established, but this has had to be kept under constant discussion. The re-drawing of the map of Europe after the recent dramatic events within Central and Eastern Europe has ensured that the notion of a wider Europe is kept firmly on the agenda.

The European Parliament and the Commission have endeavoured to ensure that the programme that they pursue is not only about improving business and trade. The market should be balanced by a social dimension going beyond health and safety issues to provide both protection and participation for all, given the new opportunities and mobility opened up by the programme since 1992. The overall aim is to underpin basic principles such as workers' rights to fair wages, to adequate social protection, to freedom of association and collective bargaining, as well as improving working conditions and vocational training. The social dimension of the European Community also embraces the rights of the young, the disabled and the elderly. In the single market the transferability of social security, pension and health care rights becomes vitally important. The Community is working towards this as part of its objective. Special programmes have been embarked upon in order to help fight the effects of cancer, AIDS, drugs misuse and environmental safety. The Community has promoted scientific research since its inception. Various areas of research are covered, including information technology, energy, industrial technologies and telecommunications. All of the projects involve partners in two or more member states. The Community's education programmes are concerned with Europe's human potential. Programmes include those which aim to link higher education with industry to improve training in new technologies and these are designed to promote mobility in higher education.

The Community works in partnership with international organisations such as the World Health Organisation, the United Nations, the Red Cross and many voluntary aid organisations within its own member states. It is a dynamic organisation and has more than doubled its size since its foundation some 40 years ago. The increasing areas of economic, social and political concern which are handled at European level and regulated by EEC law are indications of the readiness of member states to work together, where this is a logical and beneficial aspect within the Union.

So what are the implications of any forthcoming initiatives and the need for cooperation amongst the professions? The initiatives which herald the way for change and which emanate from activity in the European Community have in some respects brought about reforms that have fractured previous professional organisational structures, and in turn have demanded a change in the way professions function and also a change in the values which they may have previously held.

The changes which ensue may well bring about different views when professional groups come into contact when trying to achieve some of the international objectives for health and social care. In turn this may contribute to a breakdown of stereotyped attitudes and defensiveness amongst the professions. It is increasingly the case that programme planners working within the domain of vocational training and education consider the following as important in the predicted outcomes of the European impact:

● The reciprocity of learning from experience of others who are engaged in meeting the challenge of similar health and social problems.

- The impact that economic policies have on the quality of life standards of ordinary citizens.
- The resultant worker mobility within Europe is likely to identify problems which can only be overcome with assistance from their home country.
- An increasing number of professionals who wish to exercise their right to practise their trade, occupation or profession in other countries.
- Comparative visits and human resource exchange between practitioners, teachers and students will become increasingly common
- The European legal effects, the conventions and policies will have a growing impact on the service users and professionals in the contributing countries.

A number of these factors do of course have clear implications for the professions. For example the removal of technical barriers which includes the mutual recognition of qualifications. This means that within certain criteria the qualifications thought to be necessary to pursue a particular profession will be recognised in the member states. The professionals will need to collaborate effectively with the objective of reducing the gap between the advantaged and the weaker areas of the Community.

EUROPEAN VOCATIONAL TRAINING

Article 118 of the Treaty of Rome states that the Commission has the responsibility to promote cooperation between member States in the area of basic and advanced vocational training. Further on in this particular Treaty, article 128 states that the Community can lay down general principles for implementing a common vocational training policy. It is interesting to note that the legal framework of the European Community in the field of vocational training is interpreted in such a way that it includes the whole of higher education. Effective collaboration and cooperation between the professions will enable the development of the field of education and training as it applies to European perspectives to be achieved by effective joint working rather than by attempting to harmonise or standardise the systems of vocational preparation or professional practice. It is becoming increasingly accepted that the need to learn from each other and to work together to develop a European dimension as it relates to education has to be fostered continuously in an open and mature way by the professions.

In the area of vocational training, the European Commission is responsible for the instigation and implementation of programmes in support of member states· policies; for the purpose of these programmes the whole of higher education is viewed as vocational training. In the field of more general education the Commissioner's role is confined to the coordination of intergovernmental cooperation (Preston, 1991).

There is a task force which covers human resources, education, training and youth. It is responsible for the overall development of the major education and training programmes. It has a direct line of responsibility to the Commissioner of the European Community and sees itself as an enabler by assisting the member states to overcome some of the problems facing this sector. It also encourages people across the community to work together. It does this by drawing strength from the variety of education and training systems found throughout the member states. There are five functional units within the task force and these are:

- Cooperation in education;
- Industry–University cooperation in high technology (this is also concerned with training in central and eastern Europe);
- Education and training for technological change ;
- Initial and continuous training in vocational qualifications;
- Strategic planning, evaluation and links with other community programmes.

The process of policy-making within the Commission has a wide network and expertise to draw upon; for example in vocational training, the advisory committee has 70 members representing governments, employers and trade unions. For each of the major vocational training programmes the Commission has established either a management or an advisory committee. The effects of all these types of initiatives are now being felt within the arena of professional preparation, education and training. This can be seen by examining the Education Council's five objectives which were formulated in 1989 and which were aimed to take effect up to 1993 and beyond. Briefly these can be described as:

1. A multicultural Europe will be promoted via a European dimension in education which is to include the concept of multilingualism.
2. A mobile Europe; this will be aimed at encouraging student and tutor exchanges at all levels and enhancing the principle of mutual recognition of qualifications.
3. Training for all in Europe. This will offer equal opportunities and equality of training and education access, thereby assisting in the reduction of scholastic failure.
4. A Europe of skills, through sound basic and continuing education and training which will enable teachers to adapt to change.
5. A Europe accessible to the world; through collaboration with international educational organisations and reinforced links with non-EEC countries, lesser-developed countries especially those in central and eastern Europe will benefit.

The vocational training initiatives which have been promulgated in the European Community are likely to continue to grow apace in the immediate future. An example of this is the memorandum which the Commission issued in 1990 on the rationalisation of community vocational training programmes, COM(90). This important memorandum aimed to establish an overall framework for all community initiatives in the area of vocational training. A specific objective of the rationalisation is to design general objectives for the whole sector, thereby bringing greater coherence to the management of programmes within each State. Most of the existing vocational training programmes were scheduled to run until 1994, so the Commissioners' proposals for rationalisation are likely to be issued over the next 3 years now that they have been determined. So it is likely that as we move towards the effects of a single European Act it will be possible for the professions to see that the physical and technical barriers which have hitherto acted to impede progress may be eliminated in order to create an arena without internal frontiers, in which the free movement of persons, services and capital is assured.

All of this political and intense activity may seem remote initially to those working in direct service provision, but of course it isn't. The contributing nations face many of the same contemporary social problems such as immuno-suppressive diseases, cancers, an ageing population, child abuse, abuse of elders, racism and chronic unemployment. We have a lot to learn from each other and to share with each other in the way these negative influences are tackled. The encouragement of travel and comparative study can help professionals to see policies and practices in their own country in a different light, and to formulate questions and design solutions which may assist them to help those in most need. The upturn in employment in some contributing communities has seen high levels of prosperity in comparison to what they may have had three decades ago. This has also carried with it the additional stresses of rural de-population and intense urban living. Traditional values and beliefs can become threatened and support systems destroyed in these circumstances. Social care agencies often find themselves in a position of being forced to respond to unpredictable consequences of what is sometimes seen at first to be progress and prosperity.

The predicament which the mobility of populations is bringing about makes consequent demands upon both health and social care services. It therefore makes sense that they have to learn new ways of working as new markets are opened. The way they respond to the demands will be important but it will not be easy, there are differences in language, cultures and religions and these all make for increasing complexity. European Community declarations, charters, directives, treaties and case-law carry increasing implications. Professionals are very often not able to show evidence of even beginning to understand these implications. But in the future they will have to be alive to the European activities and innovations.

THE WORLD HEALTH ORGANISATION – THE DIMENSIONS OF HEALTH TARGETS

The World Health Organisation is a specialised agency of the United Nations with a primary responsibility for international health matters and public health. Through this organisation, created in 1948, the health professions of some 165 countries exchange their knowledge and experience with the aim of attaining a level of health for all citizens of the world, by the year 2000, that will permit them to lead a socially and economically productive life.

The European region embraces some 850 000 000 people in an area stretching from Greenland in the north and the Mediterranean in the south to the Pacific shores of Russia. It is unique in that a large proportion of its countries are industrialised with advanced medical services. Therefore the European programme of the World Health Organisation differs from that of other regions as it con-

211

centrates on the problems associated with industrial society. Much of the policy that is being created on a national basis in contributing states has its roots in the strategy of the World Health Organisation of *Health for All by the Year 2000*. Once again professions are being pushed towards effective collaboration in order for these targets to be a reality. Indeed, the demands on these professions will become greater as the three main areas of activities associated with *Health for All* are pursued. These are:

- The promotion of lifestyles conducive to health;
- Reduction of preventable conditions; and
- Provision of care that is adequate, accessible and acceptable to all.

The broad perspective of the *Health for All* policy for Europe, which consists of 38 targets, means that it is of paramount importance that the contributing professions work together in achieving the overall aims. No one profession has the franchise on the raising of the health status of any nation, and of course it becomes futile to consider health issues in isolation from the social, educational and economic activities which are associated with the broader concept of health.

In summary, the health policy for Europe addresses 3 main areas:

- The improvements in health status which are expected over the 20 year period from 1980 to the year 2000;
- The changes in lifestyles, improvements in the environment and the developments in the prevention, treatment, care and rehabilitation that will make it possible to attain the targets;
- Policy formulation and sustained implementation on the basis of political, managerial and institutional support and coordination.

The outcomes that the *Health for All* movement in the European region strives to achieve are composed of four dimensions:

1. Ensuring equity in health by reducing disparities in health status between countries and between groups within countries;
2. Adding a life to years by helping people to achieve and use their full physical, mental and social potential;
3. Adding health to life by reducing disease and disability;
4. Adding years to life by increasing life expectancy.

212

Of all the strategies available for achieving such aims, which include healthier lifestyles and improvements in the environment, it is the provision of high-quality services for prevention, treatment, care and rehabilitation that is likely to be most effective. The targets have been to a large extent successful in meeting their intention to fuel the debate on the formulation of national health policies, together with how these have been implemented in member states.

Since the first European *Health for All* policy and target statements were adopted in 1984, significant changes have taken place in Europe. The overall population has grown older and there have been positive and negative changes in the health status of the population and its determinants. Concern about the environment and its effects on health has grown rapidly. Unprecedented political and economic developments have occurred in central and eastern Europe, whilst the trend towards integration amongst other European member states has continued.

There are six major themes which have been identified by the WHO in their summary document (WHO, 1991). The themes are important to professionals and certainly send clear messages regarding the implications for cooperation amongst professions. Consider the following:

1. *Equity is the essence of Health for All*
   This concept means that all people should have a fair opportunity to realise their full health potential. This means that professions need to harmonise their activities in order that policies work effectively in improving the living and working conditions of the disadvantaged. This has to occur in order to raise the standards of their physical and social environment to levels which are closer to those of their more fortunate peers. These policies mean that there should be equal access to health services.

2. *The promotion of health and the prevention of disease are important strategic issues in the Policy of Health for All*
   It is the intention to ensure that people can make full use of their physical, mental and social capacities in order to give them a positive sense of health. Professions have a role to play in reflecting the promotion of positive lifestyles and the building of health – supportive environments and the re-configuration of health services – in order that they can deliver high quality care in effective and efficient ways.

213

3. *People themselves will achieve Health for All*
   Professionals as practitioners have a functional duty to keep the population well-informed and motivated so that they can participate actively in setting their priorities and in making and carrying out decisions. Similarly, effective teamworking which has been described earlier in this book should make the best use of existing human resources and, within the context of *Health for All*, strengthen individual self-esteem and self-knowledge in order to provide accurate social support.
4. *Many sectors of society must collaborate in order to achieve Health for All*
   The World Health Organisation recognises that intersectoral participation is needed to ensure health and protection from risks in the physical, economic and social environment. The ways in which professionals function have implications for the way in which government agencies cooperate at national, regional and local levels. It also implies a constant search for quality as well as cooperation between business and industry, labour relations and other practitioner groups.
5. *A harmonious Health Service system focuses on primary health care and adequate referral services and provides affordable, quality care*
   This means that professionals have to play their part in ensuring that the basic health needs of each community are met through services which are located as close as possible to where people live and work. They should be easily accessible, provide quality care, and involve the community in the management of complimentary, public, private and voluntary or independent health and social care institutions.
6. *An increasing number of health problems transcend national frontiers*
   Strong international cooperation, which rests heavily upon the duty of care by the professions, makes it possible to ensure environmental protection, access to adequate resources for healthy living, together with the provision of care that is of high quality and takes the best advantage of current knowledge, skills and technology.

Since the adoption of the original regional *Health for All* targets in 1984, political developments have had profound effects on the social fabric and the conduct of public affairs in all parts of the European region (WHO, 1991). The continuing influence of political and economic changes in the countries of central and eastern Europe together with the integration in western and southern Europe will obviously necessitate strong cooperation, openness and flexibility. The significant changes and contemporary trends in Europe mean that the fundamentals of the European *Health for All* strategy remain as relevant as we move to the next millennium as they are now. The magnitude of the task of attaining a *Health for All*, means that not only a strong political will and the promotion of public support are important, but that cooperation and collaboration of professions associated with health and social care are of fundamental importance for ensuring that action is taken to make the ideal become a reality. Just as the process of sustaining and mobilising further support should be seen as a responsibility at the highest level in all sectors throughout each country, this in turn is echoed in the way in which practitioners are expected to function in the future.

The *Health for All* targets are identified in the following pages and hopefully it can be seen that the topics contained in other chapters in this book are intended to assist in reflecting the underpinning elements of these targets, together with helping professionals to anticipate and respond in a competent way with the intention of enhancing their function.

THE ACHIEVEMENT OF BETTER HEALTH: *HEALTH FOR ALL* TARGETS

Targets 1–12 seek to identify the application of the *Health for All* strategy in the European region. They express in specific and often quantifiable terms the improvements in health status which are expected over the coming years up to the year 2000. Targets 1–12 fall into three categories. Two are concerned with basic policy orientation of the European strategy towards equity and wider attainment of the health potential. Four are concerned with the health of particular population groups, namely children and young people, women, the elderly and people with disabilities; their purpose is to encourage comprehensive policies and strategies to address the wide range of health issues that concern those groups. The remaining six targets are concerned with preventing the morbidity, disability and mortality associated with communicable and non-communicable diseases, accidents, mental disorders and suicides.

It is possible to identify how groups of individuals and organisations, particularly those associated with professional practice, could work together in forming 'healthy alliances' in order to promote and achieve the targets. The successful attainment of the objectives of interdisciplinary teamwork could facilitate this.

A push to attain better health

Target 1

By the Year 2000, the differences in health status between countries and between groups within countries should be reduced by at least 25%, by improving the level of health of disadvantaged nations and groups

In order to attain the level of equity in health which this target addresses, the contribution of the interdisciplinary team should concentrate on the monitoring of differences in health status between different geographical areas and socio-economic groups. Of course this also concerns professionals seeking access to adequate health care facilities and supporting health in particular living and working environments.

Target 2

By the Year 2000 all people should have the opportunity to develop and use their own health potential in order to lead socially, economically and mentally fulfilling lives

It can be seen that this target involves the issue of quality of life, and its attainment depends upon a greater emphasis being placed on the quality of life in providing primary, secondary and tertiary care. The social services have a particular role here in relation to strengthening their own function which in turn helps the individual to actively participate in community life.

Target 3

By the Year 2000, people with disabilities should be able to lead socially, economically and mentally fulfilling lives with support of special arrangements that improve their physical, social and economic opportunities

It can be seen that in order to provide better opportunities for those people with disabilities, interprofessional teamwork is of particular value, not least in promoting positive attitudes and creating non-handicapping environments for people with disabilities. Fortunately, it is possible for professionals to work together in order to provide appropriate services and support to those who do not have the ability to remain independent.

Target 4

By the Year 2000 there should be a sustained and continued reduction in morbidity and disability due to chronic disease in the region

It is hoped that this target can be attained through a reduction of at least 10 per cent in morbidity and disability due to chronic disease. In order to achieve this, a strategy will require to be adopted which operates on common risk factors and concentrates on integrating interventions within different sectors of the community.

Target 5

By the Year 2000 there should be no indigenous cases of poliomyelitis, diphtheria, neonatal tetanus, measles, mumps and congenital rubella in the region and there should be sustained and continued reduction in the incidence and adverse consequences of other communicable diseases, notably HIV infection

The major interdisciplinary effort in relation to this target means focused work in order to control strategies implemented through well-organised health care systems, which in turn ensures effective epidemiological surveillance, education, treatment and care. This is particularly well portrayed when considering the need to reduce the rate of transmission of HIV infection, and therefore eleviating its negative consequences including the social reactions to people with HIV infection and AIDS.

Target 6

By the Year 2000 life expectancy at birth in the region should be at least 75 years and there should be a sustained and continuing improvement in the health of all people aged 65 years and over

Interdisciplinary work should assist in the formation of strategies which encourage a full and active participation of the elderly in community life, together with providing appropriate services and support to elderly people in need.

Target 7

This target concerns the health of children and young people.
By the Year 2000, the health of all children and young people

217

should be improved, giving them the opportunity to grow and
develop to their full physical, mental and social potential
The way in which this is likely to affect the future competence
requirements of the various disciplines may be centred upon the
protection of children as vulnerable members of society. Further,
it means encouraging skills in order that professionals work
together to ensure social, economic and psychological support
for disadvantaged children, including those with long-term illness
and disability, and for their families.

Target 8

By the Year 2000 there should be sustained and continued improve-
ment in the health of all women
One of the major aims of achieving this target is to concentrate
upon a substantial reduction in health problems of women
related to their socio-economic status and the burden of their
multiple roles. Another important feature here is a substantial
reduction in the incidence and adverse health consequences of
sexual harassment, domestic violence and rape. Professionals
assist in this process by implementing strategies that make
significant changes in the social environment and in lifestyle
patterns.

Target 9

By the Year 2000, mortality from diseases of the circulatory system
should be reduced, in the case of people under 65 years by at least
15%, and there should be progress in improving the quality of life of
all people suffering from cardio-vascular disease
This target can be attained by ensuring that health and social care
professionals implement preventative measures, acceptable to the
population, that aim at reducing the levels of major risk factors
such as smoking, hypertension, overweight and sedentary lifestyles. It also means that professionals need strategies for providing physical, psychological and social rehabilitation for people
with signs of cardiovascular disease.

Target 10

By the Year 2000, mortality from cancer in people under 65 years
should be reduced by at least 15% and the quality of life of all
people with cancer should be significantly improved
A major feature of attaining this target is making sure that the
best interdisciplinary knowledge in diagnosis, treatment, rehabi-

litation and palliative care is applied in the most effective and appropriate way.

Target 11

By the Year 2000, injury, disability and death arising from accidents should be reduced by at least 25%
The attainment of this target highlights the wide range of effort that is required, and includes joint action by the health, social, education, transport and law, engineering and industrial sectors to reduce accidents related to traffic, home, work, sports and leisure. It also tests the ability of professionals to respond rapidly to needs that arise during emergencies and disasters and their aftermath.

Target 12

This is concerned with the reduction in mental disorders and suicides.

By the Year 2000, there should be a sustained and continuing reduction in the prevalence of mental disorders, an improvement in the quality of life of all people with such disorders, and reversal of the rising trends in suicide and attempted suicide
The way this target can be attained which is heavily dependent upon inter-disciplinary and effective teamwork includes:

- Improvement in societal factors, such as unemployment and social isolation;
- Improvement of access to measures that support people and equip them to cope with distressing or stressful events;
- Improved access to measures that support carers, both formal and informal, together with people with mental disorders;
- A greater involvement of the professions in primary health care;
- Increased efforts to prevent health threatening patterns of behaviour such as substance misuse.

Lifestyles conducive to health

The actions which address the issues of health promotion are highlighted in targets 13–17. They propose national, regional and local initiatives that actively support patterns of living associated with balanced nutrition and physical activity, together with reductions in the consumption of health damaging substances such as alcohol and tobacco. These targets focus on emphasising the requirement to change the social, economic and other factors that influence the health-related choices made by individuals, groups and communities.

Target 13
The area of health and public policy.
Introducing mechanisms at local and regional levels to involve people in policy-making and implementation.

Target 14 addresses the settings for health promotion and it requires a fostering and strengthening of cooperation to create better opportunities for healthy living, together with facilitating community participation in decisions regarding health and health promotion. It specifically looks towards the encouragement of the involvement of a variety of disciplines in such activities in order to attain its overall aim.

Target 15 focuses on health competence and in order to attain its goal it demands a wider range of lifestyle issues to be emphasised including the encouragement of personal skills, self-esteem and social support. It identifies the need for an infrastructure to offer training and education in health promotion activities to all professionals.

Target 16 continues on the theme of healthy living through the encouragement of offering and receiving social support in order to promote peoples' ability to develop and strengthen coping skills.

Target 17 identifies balanced policies and programmes with regard to the consumption and production of dependence-producing substances such as alcohol, tobacco and psycho-active drugs.

Healthy environment

Targets 18–25 link together the emerging commitment to environmental policies that lead to ecologically sustainable development, the prevention and control of risks and the equitable access to healthy environments. Their overall aim is to provide opportunities for people to live in communities with socially and physically supportive environments. The success in achieving these targets relies heavily upon regional and local mechanisms for involving people in policy development and implementation. The professions can be considered as primary producers and potential activists in encouraging environmental health action based on a full sharing of information.

Targets 26–31 address the provision of prevention, treatment and care services. The focus of health care revolves around locally accessible primary care, supported by secondary and tertiary activity that is all-embracing and responsive to health needs, and supplemented by services for people with special needs.

An underpinning framework for this set of targets is the effective management of human, financial and physical resources in a manner that is consistent with the development of the quality and cost effectiveness and efficiency of care. The targets range from direct health service policy in target 26 – which implores member states to state clearly the lines along which health services will develop, and stresses the need for them to be based on the principles of physical and economic accessibility, quality and cultural acceptability. All the targets in this group require the securing of the active participation of the public and health service providers in policy formulation and implementation.

Target 27 addresses the health service resources and management issues, and particularly stresses the fact that human resource practices within the health services rely on achieving teamwork which is effective to motivate and attain job satisfaction for people working within this service in the pursuit of excellence.

Target 28 is particularly important as it highlights the need for primary health care. In order to attain this target, the need to strengthen active outreach work to the community and coopera-tion with other sectors to achieve effective use of health service is reinforced. The targets attainment-focus specifically views the organisation of primary care in such a way as to achieve the integration of services based on effective interprofessional team-work amongst the providers. This is intended to reinforce the need for mutual provision of support at all levels of care.

Target 29, although focused on hospital care, recognises the need to organise care in such a way as to achieve the integration of services based on effective teamwork amongst care professionals.

Target 30 revolves around community services to meet special needs, and it is envisaged that by the year 2000, people needing long-term care and support in member states should have access to appropriate services of high quality.

This means that care services have to be developed which have been specifically designed to meet the needs of people suffering from chronic illness or from physical, mental or social disability. In turn, this means that the effective coordination of health services with social and income support services has to be acquired together with the establishment of appropriate communication systems.

Target 31 addresses the need to ensure continuous improvement in the quality of health care and the appropriate development and use of health technologies.

In order to maintain the quality of care, this target highlights the fact that it is a requirement that planners address the need to re-orientate the training of health service personnel to strengthen the emphasis on health status, quality of life, patients' satisfaction, and cost-effectiveness as performance measures.

The development strategies

All of the targets 1–31 can be seen to demand sustained political, managerial and financial support which is linked through a co-ordinated approach to policy formulation and its effective implementation. The strategic ways in which this can be achieved are considered in targets 32–38. It can be identified throughout the WHO targets that the foundation of support is the formulation of a health policy and an implementation strategy that takes a balanced approach to the areas of health, and that they rest on the strengthened political accountability at different levels.

Targets 32–38 focus on the need to inspire health development and to facilitate cooperation and community participation, manage human-resource development and improve information support within an effective code of ethics.

Target 32 specifically addresses the need for health research and development, and the way in which this can be achieved relies heavily on the strengthening of cooperation between the scientific community and decision-makers in the application of new knowledge to the *Health for All* developments.

Target 33 is focused primarily on policy development, and this is underpinned by the need for effective collaboration and specific policies aimed at continuously adapting strategies which are suitable to the political and administrative structure of the country.

Target 34 focuses on managing the development of *Health for All*. This requires effective collaboration and coordination and the ability of managers within services to define and prioritise problems based upon the assessment of populations and the prevalence of social and environmental risks in the overall evaluation of health system performance.

Target 35 highlights health information support. The contributing professions will have to provide intelligence systems in order to forecast future problems and needs. It also requires effective interprofessional communication systems in order to facilitate information exchange and to provide strategists and policy-makers with relevant information.

Target 36 highlights the development of human resources for health. The WHO emphasised in this target the need for basic and continuing education programmes for personnel to emphasise the principles and strategies of *Health for All* and their application in practice. This has a strong bearing on the future preparation of professionals, as the objectives and values are communicated to other sectors relevant to health for incorporation in their educational programmes and their practice. Further, basic and continuing education programmes are to place special emphasis on leadership development which encourages participants to become *Health for All* advocates.

Target 37
By the Year 2000, in all member states, a wide range of organisations and groups throughout the public, private and voluntary sectors should be actively contributing to the achievement of Health for All
It is recognised in this very important target that partners in the process will have to ensure that they:

- facilitate networking and communication between potential partners;
- provide access to priority-setting, planning, decision-making and implementation;
- strengthen international solidarity for European *Health for All* development by using existing and emerging European structures for cooperation within and between governments, with action directed towards the dissemination of information on health issues.

Target 38 highlights health and ethics and emphasises the need for the education and training of health professionals in ethics. It encourages the development of an ethical code of practice for health professionals which includes the relationship between care providers and service users. Finally, it highlights the need for professionals to take full account of the health-related ethical principles contained in the Universal Declaration of Human Rights, the United Nations Convention on Human Rights, the working recommendation of the United Nations Commission on Human Rights and the Recommendations of the Council of Europe.

All member states have accepted the duty and responsibility of taking the necessary action to ensure the attainment of *Health for All by the Year 2000*. This commitment logically leads to these principles being reflected in the future training programmes and management agendas for professions associated with health care. The targets are about action, partnership and innovation. Professionals have a key part to play in turning the policy and intentions into results for the people within the communities which they serve. This ensures that the achievements are of the best quality that can be attained and will assist in the reduction of unacceptable differences in the state of health of the contributing communities. The overall challenge identified by the WHO still remains, and that is to combine the different components of targets into cohesive programmes of action, each of which stimulates, involves and gives incentives to the public, private and voluntary sectors at local, national and international levels which results in progress towards the achievement of the overall goals.

One consequence of these targets is that it is likely that operational management, which characteristically thinks in terms of days or weeks ahead at local level, and strategic management, which may think in terms of years ahead on a regional or global basis, will need to consider the factors associated with the targets as they affect their areas of work.

The competencies required to achieve such aims as are identified in the WHO framework are those which are associated with working together and being inter-functional rather than job specific on some occasions. These might for example include the strengthening of communication competencies. All professions must face the challenge of constant change. To do so successfully, health and social care organisations must find ways to raise the level of competence of their participants and in particular their managers and specialists. This means that the need for continuous professional development has to be incorporated into training and work strategies which in turn necessitates training programmes being geared to achieving the aims of well thought out global targets.

References

Commission Memorandum on the Rationalisation and Coordination of Vocational Programmes at Community Level. COM(90) 334 final, 21 August 1990) European Communities, Brussels.

Preston, J. (1991) *European Community Education Training and Research Programmes: an Action Guide*, London Kogan Page 1991.

World Health Organisation (1978) *Primary Health Care. Health for All Series No.1*. Geneva, Alma Ata (1978).

World Health Organisation (1991) *The Health Policy for Europe – Summary of the Updated Edition*, Copenhagen. WHO Regional Office for Europe.

mental disorders, WHO
targets 219
mental health needs
categories 61
measuring 60–4
national averages 61
v. resources 60
see also needs
monitoring
feedback 47–8
as supervision task 27
multidisciplinary working,
definition 187
multilingualism 210

National Council for Vocational
Qualifications (NCVQ) 105–6,
161, 183
National Vocational Qualifications
(NVQs) 109, 110
government policy 148
professionals' concern 147
NCVQ (National Council for
Vocational
Qualifications) 106, 161, 183
needs
assessment as base for team
planning 36, 38
care programmes 40–1
categorisation 39–40
differing definitions of 40
needs-related diversity 46
team operational policy 43
see also mental health needs
network teams 11, 12–13, 16
NHS and Community Care Act
(1990) 192–3
nurse dilemma 94–5
NVQs see National Vocational
Qualifications

occupational standards
development of 146–8, 160–1,
183
functional maps as starting
point 161
set by employers? 146–7, 153
see also qualifications
Occupational Standards
Councils 158–59

Care Sector Consortium 146,
147–8, 159, 179
Employment Occupational
Standards Council 150
omnipotence, myth of 1
openness, trend towards 94–5
outcomes, as measures of
effectiveness 195

parents, single, and mental
distress 62
participation see patient
participation
pathways see client pathways
patient advocates 91
patient assessment 125–6
common format for teams 97
information for patient 94–5
patient involvement in 91
patient participation
as antidote to internalising
trends 196–7
in assessment 91
auditing 98–9
balance in decision-making 88–
9
concepts and purposes 81–5
consulting 86–7
danger of generalisation 100
ideological arguments for 100–
1
increasing 89–92
information giving 85–6, 91
joint decisions 87
and multidisciplinary teams 92–
3
overview 99–101
patient decisions 87–8
therapeutic benefit 89
types of 85–8
wanted by patients? 90
patient power
effect on interprofessional
working 93–8
trends in 81–2
patient–practitioner matching 18
patient–practitioner
relationships 86–9, 93
co-service 83, 84–5
sources of change in 81–2